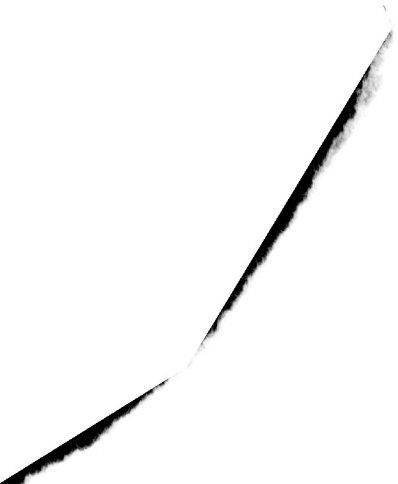

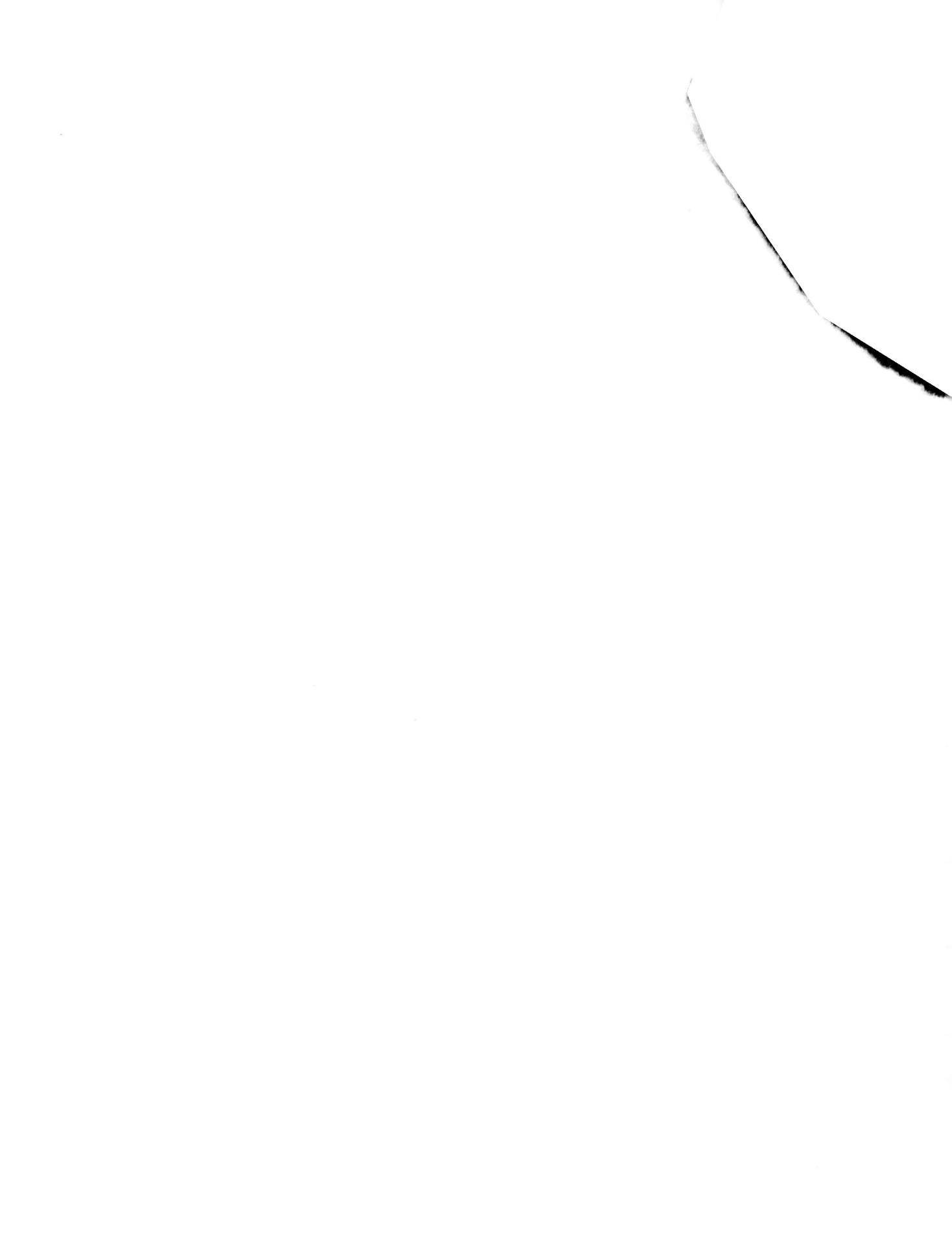

# DASH DIET for

# TWO

2 BOOKS IN 1

## Cookbook

The Best 220+ Healthy Recipes to cook with your partner! Taste yourself and your love with many heart-healthy recipes for couple!

By

Michelle Sandler

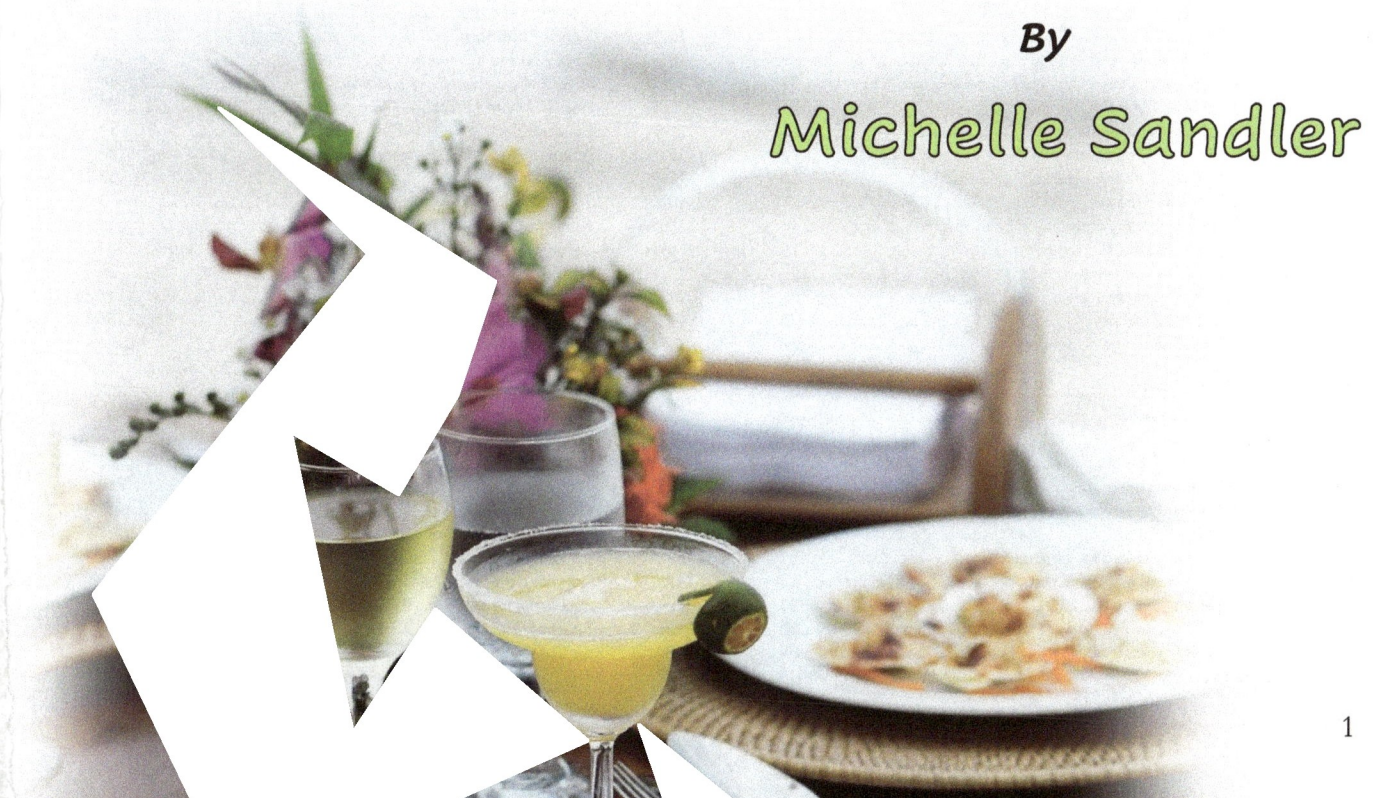

# Table of Contents

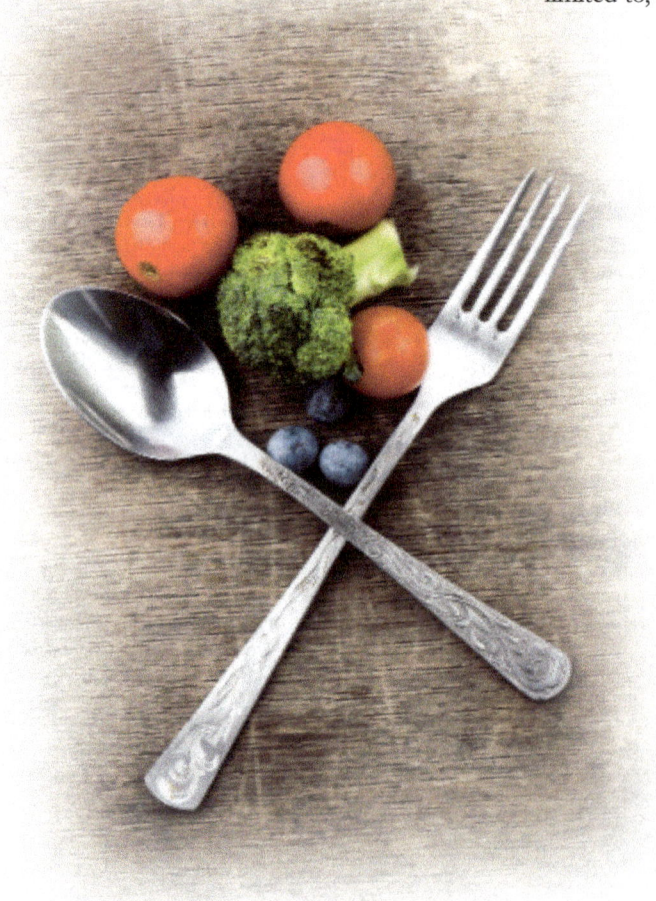

## Introduction

The DASH Diet is the perfect dietary regimen specifically for **heart health**. It is in fact one of the few diets in the world specifically designed to reduce triglycerides and bad cholesterol in the blood, in order to improve blood pressure and blood circulation.

The purpose of the DASH diet is to improve the health of all the persons who follow it. After careful clinical studies conducted in the United States, the Dash Diet is currently recommended by many medical associations in the world, especially for all of people at risk of developing cardiovascular disease.

In the Dash Diet the word **DASH** is an acronym: it stands for *Dietary Approaches to Stop Hypertension.*

Dash Diet is not related to weight loss. In fact, the number of calories introduced is equal to the daily nutritional requirements (it is a so-called isocaloric diet) and not less. However, there are some **variants of the Dash Diet** specific for overweight people, based on the consumption of the same foods but in smaller portions in order to reduce the calories acquired.

## *What are the additional benefits of following the DASH diet?*

Clinical studies show that a high consumption of fruits and vegetables reduces the risk of developing **diabetes**, **cancer, atherosclerosis**, and other diseases typical of old age.

Replacing saturated fats, found in butter or cheese, with unsaturated fats, found in nuts, olive oil, and seeds, helps reduce triglycerides and cholesterol, greatly reducing the chance of developing cardiovascular disease.

Anyone can follow the Dash Diet: **women**, **kids**, **athletes**, **older people**, **sedentary people** and **men**!

However, scientists discovered that each family member should eat in different portions and in a different way.

*How many times did you go crazy to find two or three different recipes to cook for you and your partner or family?*

I think all of us should follow this diet to have a much healthier lifestyle and live better and longer, and this is why I created this a fantastic book series about DASH Diet: *"Dash Diet for Two Cookbook"* is the first collection of this series and it was born to give all my brilliant readers the possibility to stop going crazy to find the right recipes for all family members! Indeed, *"Dash Diet for Two"* is the collection of 2 of my best books: *"The Dash Diet for Him Cookbook"* and *"The Dash diet One Cookbook"*. And, what is no better than more than 220 Dash recipes for a couple of persons who want to increase their heart health and prevent diseases!

**Dash Diet involves eating certain foods and reducing (or sometimes eliminating) others.**

## Yes foods:
- Vegetables
- Carbohydrates from whole grains
- Fruit
- Low-fat dairy products
- Fish
- White meat
- Vegetable oils
- Sea Salt/Himalayan salt

## No foods:
- Red meat
- Animal fats
- Sugar
- Alcohol
- Processed products
- Synthetic salt (sodium chloride)
- Preservatives

# BOOK 1: "THE DASH DIET FOR HIM Cookbook"

# Chapter 1.
# BREAKFAST AND SNACKS

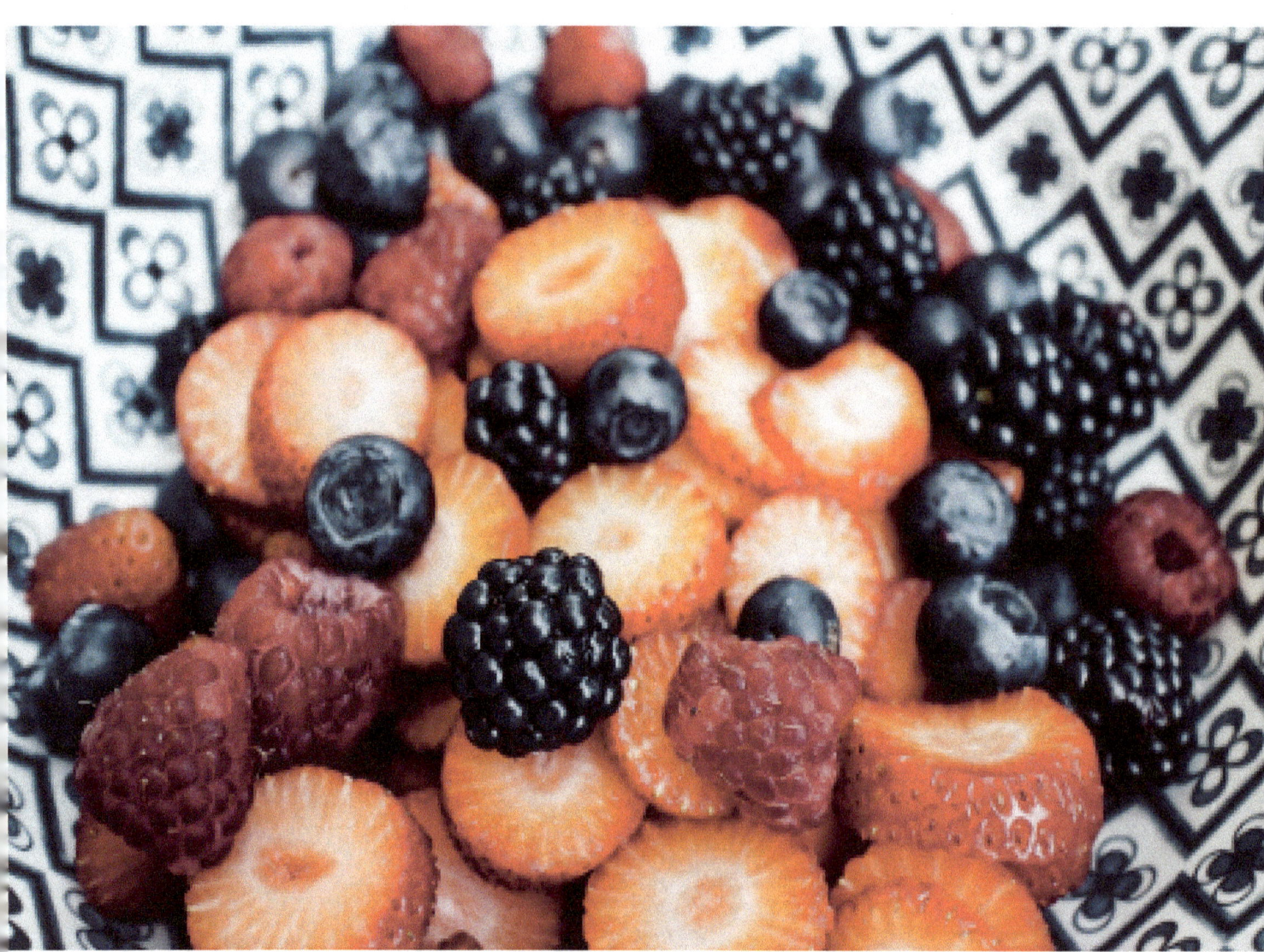

| 1) BANANA STEEL OATS | | |
|---|---|---|
| **Preparation Time**: 10 minutes | **Cooking Time:** 15 minutes | **Servings: 3** |

| Ingredients: | Ingredients: |
|---|---|
| ✓ 1 small banana<br>✓ 1 cup almond milk<br>✓ ¼ teaspoon cinnamon, ground | ✓ ½ cup rolled oats<br>✓ 1 tablespoon honey |

| Directions: | ❖ Reduce heat to medium-low and simmer for 5-7 minutes until oats are tender.<br>❖ Dice the remaining half of the banana and place on top of the oatmeal. Enjoy! |
|---|---|
| ❖ Take a casserole dish and add half of the banana, whisk in almond milk, ground cinnamon.<br>❖ Season with the sunflower seeds. Stir until the banana is well mashed, bring the mixture to a boil and stir in the oats. | |

| 2) PINEAPPLE OATMEAL | | |
|---|---|---|
| **Preparation Time**: 10 minutes | **Cooking Time:** 4-8 hours | **Servings: 5** |

| Ingredients: | Ingredients: |
|---|---|
| ✓ 1 cup steel-cut oats<br>✓ 4 cups unsweetened almond milk<br>✓ 2 medium apples, sliced<br>✓ 1 teaspoon coconut oil | ✓ 1 teaspoon cinnamon<br>✓ ¼ teaspoon nutmeg<br>✓ 2 tablespoons maple syrup, unsweetened<br>✓ A trickle of lemon juice |

| Directions: | ❖ Stir gently. Add desired toppings. Serve and enjoy!<br>❖ Store in the refrigerator for later use; be sure to add a splash of almond milk after reheating for added flavor. |
|---|---|
| ❖ Add the listed ingredients to a pot and mix well.<br>❖ Cook on very low heat for 8 hours or on high heat for 4 hours. | |

| 3) CRISPY FLAX AND ALMOND CRACKERS | | |
|---|---|---|
| **Preparation Time**: 15 minutes | **Cooking Time:** 60 minutes | **Servings: 20-24 crackers** |

| Ingredients: | Ingredients: |
|---|---|
| ✓ ½ cup ground flaxseed<br>✓ ½ cup almond flour<br>✓ 1 tablespoon coconut flour<br>✓ 2 tablespoons shelled hemp seeds | ✓ ¼ teaspoon sunflower seeds<br>✓ 1 egg white<br>✓ 2 tablespoons unsalted almond butter, melted |

| Directions: | ❖ Add egg whites and melted almond butter, mix until combined.<br>❖ Transfer dough to a sheet of parchment paper and cover with another sheet of paper.<br>❖ Roll out dough. Cut into crackers and bake for 60 minutes. Let them cool and enjoy! |
|---|---|
| ❖ Preheat oven to 300 degrees F.<br>❖ Line a baking sheet with baking paper, set aside.<br>❖ Add flax, almonds, coconut flour, hemp seeds to a bowl and mix. | |

## 4) COOL MUSHROOM MUNCHIES

| **Preparation Time**: 5 minutes | **Cooking Time**: 10 minutes | **Servings**: 2 |
| --- | --- | --- |

Ingredients:

- ✓ 4 caps Portobello mushrooms
- ✓ 3 tablespoons coconut aminos
- ✓ 2 tablespoons sesame oil

Ingredients:

- ✓ 1 tablespoon fresh ginger, minced
- ✓ 1 small clove garlic, minced

Directions:

- ❖ Set the oven to low, keeping the rack 6 inches from the heat source.
- ❖ Wash the mushrooms under cold water and transfer them to a baking sheet (top side down).

- ❖ Take a bowl and mix the sesame oil, garlic, coconut amino acid, ginger and pour the mixture over the tops of the mushrooms.
- ❖ Cook for 10 minutes. Serve and enjoy!

## 5) DELICIOUS BOWL OF QUINOA WITH BERRIES

| **Preparation Time**: 5 minutes | **Cooking Time**: 15 minutes | **Servings**: 4 |
| --- | --- | --- |

Ingredients:

- ✓ 1 cup quinoa
- ✓ 2 cups water
- ✓ 1 2-inch piece of cinnamon stick
- ✓ 2-3 tablespoons maple syrup Flavorful toppings
- ✓ ½ cup blueberries, raspberries or strawberries

Ingredients:

- ✓ 2 tablespoons raisins
- ✓ 1 teaspoon lime
- ✓ ¼ teaspoon nutmeg, grated
- ✓ 3 tablespoons whipped coconut cream
- ✓ 2 tablespoons cashews, chopped

Directions:

- ❖ Take a metal strainer and pass your grains through it to filter them well.
- ❖ Rinse the grains well under cold water.
- ❖ Take a medium sized saucepan and pour in the water.
- ❖ Add the strained grains and bring it to a boil.
- ❖ Add the cinnamon sticks and cover the saucepan.

- ❖ Lower the heat and let the mixture simmer for 15 minutes to allow the grains to absorb the liquid.
- ❖ Remove the heat and stir the mixture with a fork.
- ❖ Add maple syrup if you want additional flavor.
- ❖ Also, if you want to make things a little more interesting, just add any of the above ingredients.

## 6) BOWL OF QUINOA AND CINNAMON

| **Preparation Time**: 10 minutes | **Cooking Time**: 15 minutes | **Servings**: 2 |
| --- | --- | --- |

Ingredients:

- ✓ 1 cup uncooked quinoa
- ✓ 1½ cups water
- ✓ ½ teaspoon cinnamon powder

Ingredients:

- ✓ ½ teaspoon sunflower seeds
- ✓ A drizzle of almond/coconut milk to serve

- ❖ Rinse the quinoa well under water.
- ❖ Take a medium sized saucepan and add the quinoa, water, cinnamon and seeds.
- ❖ Stir and place over medium-high heat. Bring the mix to a boil.

- ❖ Reduce the heat to low and simmer for 10 minutes.
- ❖ Once cooked, remove from heat and allow to cool.
- ❖ Serve with a drizzle of almond or coconut milk. Enjoy!

## 7)  AMAZING AND HEALTHY BOWL OF GRANOLA

| **Preparation Time**: 5 minutes | **Cooking Time:** 25 minutes | **Servings: 6** |
|---|---|---|

| Ingredients: | Ingredients: |
|---|---|
| ✓  1 ounce oatmeal Porridge<br>✓  2 teaspoons maple syrup Cooking spray if needed<br>✓  4 medium bananas<br>✓   4 jars of Fromage Frais layered caramel<br>✓  5 ounces fresh fruit salad, such as strawberries, blueberries and raspberries | ✓  ¼ ounce pumpkin seeds<br>✓  ¼ ounce sunflower seeds<br>✓  ¼ ounce dried chia seeds<br>✓  ¼ ounce dried coconut |

| Directions: | |
|---|---|
| ❖  Preheat oven to 300 degrees F.<br>❖  Take a baking sheet and line with baking paper.<br>❖  Take a large bowl and add oats, maple syrup and seeds.<br>❖  Spread the mix on a baking sheet. | ❖  Drizzle coconut oil on top and bake for 20 minutes, making sure to keep stirring occasionally.<br>❖  Sprinkle with coconut after the first 15 minutes. Remove from oven and allow to cool.<br>❖  Take a bowl and layer sliced bananas on top of the Fromage Fraise.<br>❖  Spread the cooled granola mix on top and serve with a berry garnish. Enjoy! |

## 8)  BOWL OF QUINOA AND DATES

| **Preparation Time**: 10 minutes | **Cooking Time:** 15 minutes | **Servings: 2** |
|---|---|---|

| Ingredients: | Ingredients: |
|---|---|
| ✓  1 date, pitted and finely chopped<br>✓  ½ cup red quinoa, dried<br>✓  1 cup unsweetened almond milk | ✓  1/8 teaspoon vanilla extract<br>✓  ¼ cup fresh strawberries, hulled and sliced<br>✓  1/8 teaspoon cinnamon powder |

| Directions: | |
|---|---|
| ❖  Take a skillet and place it over low heat. | ❖  Add the quinoa, almond milk, cinnamon, and vanilla and cook for about 15 minutes,<br>❖  making sure to keep stirring occasionally.<br>❖  Garnish with the strawberries and enjoy! |

## 9)  PUMPKIN OATS

| **Preparation Time**: 5 minutes | **Cooking Time:** 8 minutes | **Servings: 3** |
|---|---|---|

| Ingredients: | Ingredients: |
|---|---|
| ✓  1 cup quick-cooking rolled oats<br>✓  ¾ cup almond milk<br>✓  ½ cup canned pumpkin puree | ✓  ¼ teaspoon pumpkin spice<br>✓  1 teaspoon cinnamon powder |

| Directions: | |
|---|---|
| ❖  Take a microwave safe bowl and add the oats, almond milk and microwave for 1-2 minutes.<br>❖  Add more almond milk if needed to reach desired consistency. | ❖  Cook for an additional 30 seconds.<br>❖  Stir in the pumpkin puree, pumpkin pie spice and ground cinnamon. Heat gently and enjoy! |

## 10) ENERGY-RICH OATMEAL

| Preparation Time: 10-15 minutes | Cooking Time: 5 minutes | Servings: 2 |
|---|---|---|

| Ingredients: | Ingredients: |
|---|---|
| ✓  ¼ cup quick-cooking oats<br>✓  ¼ cup almond milk<br>✓  2 tablespoons low-fat Greek yogurt | ✓  ¼ cup banana, mashed<br>✓  2-1/4 tablespoons flaxseed meal |
| Directions:<br><br>❖  Whisk all ingredients together in a bowl. | ❖  Transfer the bowl to your refrigerator and let sit for 15 minutes.<br>❖  Serve and enjoy! |

## 11) MOUTH WATERING CHICKEN PORRIDGE

| Preparation Time: 1 hour | Cooking Time: 10-20 minutes | Servings: 4 |
|---|---|---|

| Ingredients: | Ingredients: |
|---|---|
| ✓  1 cup jasmine rice<br>✓  1 pound steamed/cooked chicken thighs<br>✓  5 cups chicken broth | ✓  4 cups water<br>✓  1 ½ cups fresh ginger Green onions Roasted cashews |
| Directions:<br><br>❖  Put the rice in the refrigerator and let it cool 1 hour before cooking.<br>❖  Take out the rice and add it to your Robot.<br>❖  Pour in the chicken broth and water.<br>❖  Close the lid and cook in PORRIDGE mode, using your default settings and parameters. | ❖  Release pressure naturally in 10 minutes.<br>❖  Open the lid. Remove the meat from the chicken thighs and add the meat to the soup.<br>❖  Stir well in Sauté mode. Season with a little flavored vinegar and enjoy with a garnish of walnuts and onion. |

## 12) THE "PORRIDGE" OF DECISIVE APPLES

| Preparation Time: 10 minutes | Cooking Time: 5 minutes | Servings: 2 |
|---|---|---|

| Ingredients: | Ingredients: |
|---|---|
| ✓  1 large apple, peeled, pitted and grated<br>✓  1 cup unsweetened almond milk<br>✓  1 ½ tablespoons sunflower seeds | ✓  1/8 cup fresh blueberries<br>✓  ¼ teaspoon fresh vanilla bean extract |
| Directions:<br><br>❖  Take a large skillet and add the sunflower seeds, vanilla extract, almond milk, apples and stir. | ❖  Place over medium-low heat. Cook for 5 minutes, making sure to keep the mixture stirred. Transfer to a serving bowl. Serve and enjoy |

## 13) CINNAMON AND COCONUT PORRIDGE

| **Preparation Time**: 5 minutes | **Cooking Time**: 5 minutes | **Servings: 4** |
|---|---|---|

| Ingredients: | Ingredients: |
|---|---|
| ✓ 2 cups water<br>✓ 1 cup cream of coconut<br>✓ ½ cup unsweetened dry coconut, shredded<br>✓ 2 tablespoons flaxseed meal | ✓ 1 tablespoon almond butter<br>✓ 1 ½ teaspoons stevia<br>✓ 1 teaspoon cinnamon Toppings such as blueberries |

**Directions:**

❖ Add the listed ingredients to a small saucepan, stir well.
❖ Transfer the pot to the stove and place it over medium-low heat.
❖ Bring everything to a slow boil.

❖ Stir well and remove from heat.
❖ Divide the mixture into equal portions and let them rest for 10 minutes. Top with desired toppings and enjoy!

## 14) VANILLA SWEET POTATO PORRIDGE

| **Preparation Time**: 10 minutes | **Cooking Time**: 8 hours | **Servings: 5** |
|---|---|---|

| Ingredients: | Ingredients: |
|---|---|
| ✓ 6 sweet potatoes, peeled and cut into<br>✓ 1-inch cubes<br>✓ 1 ½ cups light coconut milk<br>✓ 1 teaspoon cinnamon powder | ✓ 1 teaspoon cardamom powder<br>✓ 1 teaspoon pure vanilla extract<br>✓ 1 cup raisins Pinch of salt |

**Directions:**

❖ Add the sweet potatoes, coconut milk, vanilla, cardamom and cinnamon to your Slow Cooker.
❖ Close the lid and cook on LOW for 8 hours.

❖ Open the lid and mash all the mixture using a potato masher to mash the sweet potatoes, mix well.
❖ Add the raisins, salt and serve. Serve and enjoy!

## 15) BANANA OATMEAL VERY NUTRITIOUS

| **Preparation Time**: 15 minutes | **Cooking Time**: 7-9 hours | **Servings: 4** |
|---|---|---|

| Ingredients: | Ingredients: |
|---|---|
| ✓ 1 cup steel-cut oats<br>✓ 1 ripe banana, mashed<br>✓ 2 cups unsweetened almond milk<br>✓ 1 cup water<br>✓ 1 ½ tablespoons honey | ✓ ½ teaspoon vanilla extract<br>✓ ¼ cup almonds, chopped<br>✓ 1 teaspoon cinnamon powder<br>✓ ¼ teaspoon nutmeg powder |

**Directions:**

❖ Grease the pressure cooker well.
❖ Add the listed ingredients to the pressure cooker and stir.

❖ Cover with lid and cook on LOW for 7-9 hours. Serve and enjoy!

## 16) PERFECT HOMEMADE PICKLED GINGER GARI

| **Preparation Time**: 40 minutes | **Cooking Time:** 5 minutes | **Servings: 8** |
|---|---|---|

Ingredients:

✓ Approximately 8 ounces fresh ginger root, fully peeled
✓ 1 teaspoon and extra
✓ ½ teaspoon fine sunflower seeds

Ingredients:

✓ 1 cup vinegar, rice
✓ 1/3 cup sugar, white

Directions:

❖ Cut ginger into small pieces and transfer to a bowl.
❖ Season with sunflower seeds and stir, let the mixture sit for at least 30 minutes.
❖ Take a saucepan and add the sugar and vinegar, heat, bring the mixture to a boil and continue to boil until the sugar has completely dissolved.

❖ Pour the liquid over the ginger pieces.
❖ Let cool and wait for the water to change color. Enjoy! Alternatively, store in jars and use as needed.

## 17) HEALTHY SAUTÉED ZUCCHINI

| **Preparation Time**: 10 minutes | **Cooking Time:** 10 minutes | **Servings: 4** |
|---|---|---|

Ingredients:

✓ 2 heaped tablespoons olive oil
✓ 1 medium onion, thinly sliced
✓ 2 medium zucchini, cut into thin strips

Ingredients:

✓ 2 heaped tablespoons teriyaki sauce, low sodium
✓ 1 tablespoon coconut aminos
✓ 1 tablespoon sesame seeds, toasted Ground pepper (black) as needed

Directions:

❖ Take a skillet and place it on the stove on medium level.
❖ Add the onions and stir for 5 minutes.
❖ Add the zucchini and stir for 1 more minute.

❖ Gently add the sauces along with the sesame seeds.
❖ Cook for another 5 minutes until the zucchini is soft.
❖ Finally, add the pepper and enjoy!

## 18) INCREDIBLE SCRAMBLED TURKEY EGGS

| **Preparation Time**: 15 minutes | **Cooking Time:** 15 minutes | **Servings: 2** |
|---|---|---|

Ingredients:

✓ 1 tablespoon coconut oil
✓ 1 medium red bell pepper, diced
✓ ½ medium yellow onion, diced
✓ ¼ teaspoon chili sauce

Ingredients:

✓ 3 large free-range eggs
✓ ¼ teaspoon black pepper, freshly ground
✓ ¼ teaspoon salt

❖ Place a skillet over medium-high heat, add the coconut oil and let it heat up.
❖ Add the onions and sauté.
❖ Add the turkey and red bell bell pepper.

❖ Cook until the turkey is cooked through. Take a bowl and beat the eggs, stir in salt and pepper.
❖ Pour the eggs into the pan with the turkey and gently cook and scramble the eggs.
❖ Add the hot sauce and enjoy!

## 19) SPICY SALAMI OMELETTE

| **Preparation Time**: 5 minutes | **Cooking Time**: 20 minutes | **Servings: 2** |
| --- | --- | --- |

Ingredients:

- ✓ 3 eggs
- ✓ 7 slices of pepperoni
- ✓ 1 teaspoon of coconut cream

Ingredients:

- ✓ Salt and freshly ground black pepper, to taste
- ✓ 1 tablespoon of butter

Directions:

- ❖ Take a bowl and beat the eggs with all the remaining ingredients.
- ❖ Then take a skillet and heat the butter. Pour ¼ of the egg mixture into the pan.
- ❖ After that, cook for 2 minutes on each side.
- ❖ Repeat to use the entire batter. Serve hot and enjoy!

## 20) OMELETTE WITH HERBS AND AVOCADO

| **Preparation Time**: 2 minutes | **Cooking Time**: 10 minutes | **Servings: 2** |
| --- | --- | --- |

Ingredients:

- ✓ 3 large free-range eggs
- ✓ ½ medium avocado, sliced

Ingredients:

- ✓ ½ cup almonds, sliced Salt and pepper to taste

Directions:

- ❖ Take a non-stick skillet and place it over medium-high heat.
- ❖ Take a bowl and add the eggs, beat the eggs. Pour into the skillet and cook for 1 minute.
- ❖ Reduce the heat to low and cook for 4 minutes. Top the omelet with the almonds and avocado.
- ❖ Sprinkle with salt and pepper and serve. Enjoy!

## 21) CARROT AND ZUCCHINI OATMEAL

| **Preparation Time**: 10 minutes | **Cooking Time**: 8 hours | **Servings: 3** |
| --- | --- | --- |

Ingredients:

- ✓ ½ cup steel-cut oats
- ✓ 1 cup coconut milk
- ✓ 1 carrot, grated
- ✓ ¼ cup zucchini, grated

Ingredients:

- ✓ A pinch of nutmeg
- ✓ ½ teaspoon cinnamon powder
- ✓ 2 tablespoons brown sugar
- ✓ ¼ cup pecans, chopped

Directions:

- ❖ Grease Slow Cooker pot well.
- ❖ Add oats, zucchini, milk, carrot, nutmeg, cloves, sugar, cinnamon and mix well.
- ❖ Place lid on and cook on LOW for 8 hours.
- ❖ Divide between serving bowls and enjoy!

# chapter 2.  LUNCH

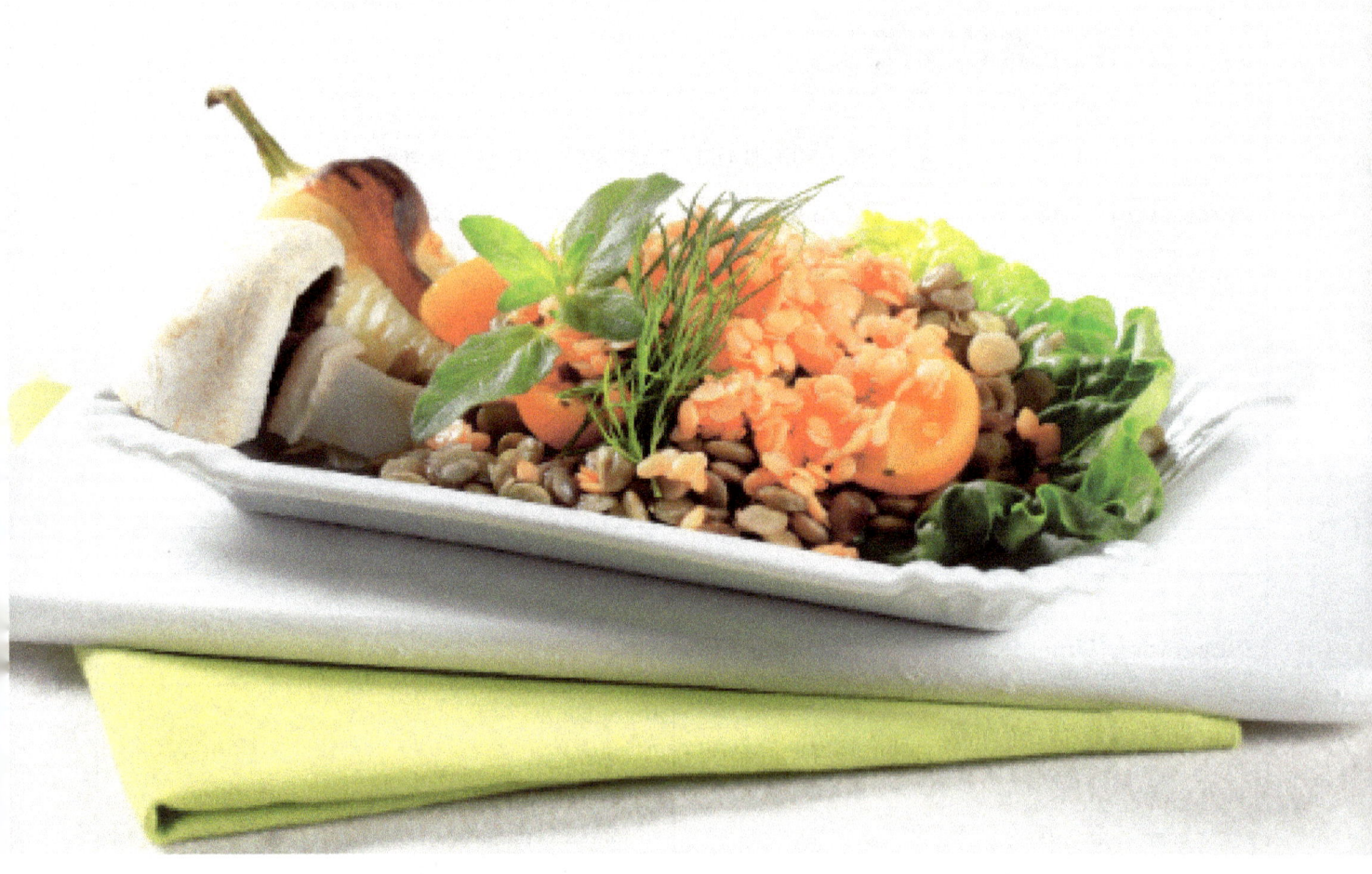

## 22) FANTASTIC MANGO CHICKEN

| **Preparation Time**: 25 minutes | **Cooking Time:** 10 minutes | **Servings: 4** |
|---|---|---|

Ingredients:

- ✓ 2 medium mangoes, peeled and chopped 10 ounces coconut milk 4 teaspoons vegetable oil 4 teaspoons spicy curry paste 14 ounces boneless,

Ingredients:

- ✓ skinless chicken breast, diced 4 medium shallots 1 large English cucumber, sliced and seeded

Directions:

- ❖ Slice half of the mangoes and add the halves to a bowl. Add the mangoes and almond and coconut milk to a blender and blend until smooth. Keep the mixture aside. Take a large pot and place it on a medium heat, add the oil and let the oil heat up.

- ❖ Add the curry paste and cook for 1 minute until fragrant, add the shallots and chicken to the pot and cook for 5 minutes. Pour in the mango puree and let it heat through. Serve the cooked chicken with the mango puree and cucumbers. Enjoy

## 23) CHICKEN LIVER STEW

| **Preparation Time**: 10 minutes | **Cooking Time:** Zero | **Servings: 2** |
|---|---|---|

Ingredients:

- ✓ 10 ounces chicken livers
- ✓ 1 ounce onion, chopped

Ingredients:

- ✓ 2 ounces sour cream
- ✓ 1 tablespoon olive oil Sunflower seeds to taste

Directions:

- ❖ Take a frying pan and place it over medium heat.
- ❖ Add the oil and let it heat up.
- ❖ Add the onions and sauté until just golden brown. Add the livers and season with the sunflower seeds.

- ❖ Cook until the livers are halfway cooked.
- ❖ Transfer the mixture to a stew pot.
- ❖ Add the sour cream and cook for 20 minutes. Serve and enjoy!

## 24) CHICKEN WITH MUSTARD

| **Preparation Time**: 10 minutes | **Cooking Time:** 40 minutes | **Servings: 2** |
|---|---|---|

Ingredients:

- ✓ 2 chicken breasts
- ✓ 1/4 cup chicken broth
- ✓ 2 tablespoons mustard
- ✓ 1 1/2 tablespoons olive oil

Ingredients:

- ✓ 1/2 teaspoon paprika
- ✓ 1/2 teaspoon chili powder
- ✓ 1/2 teaspoon garlic powder

Directions:

- ❖ Take a small bowl and mix the mustard, olive oil, paprika, chicken broth, garlic powder, chicken broth and chili.
- ❖ Add the chicken breast and marinate for 30 minutes.

- ❖ Take a lined baking sheet and arrange the chicken.
- ❖ Bake for 35 minutes at 375 degrees F. Serve and enjoy!

## 25) THE DELICIOUS TURKEY WRAP

| **Preparation Time**: 10 minutes | **Cooking Time**: 10 minutes | **Servings: 6** |
| --- | --- | --- |

Ingredients:

- 1 ¼ pounds ground turkey, lean
- 4 green onions, chopped
- 1 tablespoon olive oil
- 1 clove garlic, minced
- 2 teaspoons chili paste
- 8 ounces water chestnuts, diced

Ingredients:

- 3 tablespoons hoisin sauce
- 2 tablespoons coconut aminos
- 1 tablespoon rice vinegar
- 12 almond butter lettuce leaves
- 1/8 teaspoon sunflower seeds

Directions:

- ❖ Take a skillet and place it over medium heat, add the turkey and garlic to the pan.
- ❖ Heat for 6 minutes until cooked through.
- ❖ Take a bowl and transfer the turkey to it.

- ❖ Add the onions and water chestnuts.
- ❖ Stir in the hoisin sauce, coconut amino acid, vinegar and chili paste.
- ❖ Mix well and transfer to lettuce leaves. Serve and enjoy!

## 26) ZUCCHINI ZOODLES WITH CHICKEN AND BASIL

| **Preparation Time**: 10 minutes | **Cooking Time**: 10 minutes | **Servings: 3** |
| --- | --- | --- |

Ingredients:

- 2 chicken fillets, diced
- 2 tablespoons ghee
- 1 pound tomatoes, diced
- ½ cup basil, chopped

Ingredients:

- ¼ cup almond milk
- 1 garlic clove, peeled, chopped
- 1 zucchini, chopped

Directions:

- ❖ Fry the diced chicken in the ghee until no longer pink.
- ❖ Add the tomatoes and season with the sunflower seeds.
- ❖ Simmer and reduce the liquid.

- ❖ Prepare the Zoodles by shredding the zucchini in a food processor.
- ❖ Add the basil, garlic, coconut and almond milk to the chicken and cook for a few minutes.
- ❖ Add half of the Zucchini Zoodles to a bowl and top with the creamy tomato basil chicken. Enjoy!

## 27) BAKED CHICKEN WITH PARMESAN CHEESE

| **Preparation Time**: 5 minutes | **Cooking Time**: 20 minutes | **Servings: 2** |
| --- | --- | --- |

Ingredients:

- 2 tablespoons ghee
- 2 boneless chicken breasts, skinless Pink sunflower seeds Freshly ground black pepper
- ½ cup mayonnaise, low-fat

Ingredients:

- ¼ cup Parmesan cheese, grated
- 1 tablespoon dry Italian seasoning, low-fat, low-sodium
- ¼ cup crushed pork rind

- ❖ Preheat oven to 425 degrees F. Take a large baking sheet and coat with ghee.
- ❖ Pat the chicken breasts dry and wrap with a towel. Season with sunflower seeds and pepper.
- ❖ Place in the baking dish.

- ❖ Take a small bowl and add the mayonnaise, parmesan cheese and Italian seasoning.
- ❖ Spread mayonnaise mixture evenly over chicken breast. Sprinkle with crushed pork rind.
- ❖ Bake for 20 minutes until the topping is golden brown. Serve and enjoy!

| 28) CRAZY JAPANESE POTATO AND BEEF CROQUETTES | | |
|---|---|---|
| **Preparation Time**: 10 minutes | **Cooking Time**: 20 minutes | **Servings: 10** |

Ingredients:

- ✓ 3 medium russet potatoes, peeled and chopped
- ✓ 1 tablespoon almond butter
- ✓ 1 tablespoon vegetable oil
- ✓ 3 onions, diced

Ingredients:

- ✓ ¾ pound ground beef
- ✓ 4 teaspoons light coconut aminos All-purpose flour for coating
- ✓ 2 eggs, beaten Panko bread crumbs for coating
- ✓ ½ cup oil for frying

Directions:

- ❖ Take a saucepan and place it over medium-high heat; add the potatoes and sunflower seed water, boil for 16 minutes.
- ❖ Remove the water and place the potatoes in another bowl, add the almond butter and mash the potatoes.
- ❖ Take a frying pan and put it on medium heat, add 1 tablespoon of oil and let it heat up.
- ❖ Add the onions and sauté until tender. Add the beef coconut aminos to the onions.

- ❖ Continue frying until the beef is browned. Mix the beef with the potatoes evenly.
- ❖ Take another skillet and place it over medium heat; add half a cup of oil.
- ❖ Form croquettes with the mashed potato mixture and coat with flour, then egg and finally breadcrumbs.
- ❖ Fry the croquettes until golden brown on all sides. Enjoy!

| 29) GOLDEN EGGPLANT CHIPS | | |
|---|---|---|
| **Preparation Time**: 10 minutes | **Cooking Time**: 15 minutes | **Servings: 8** |

Ingredients:

- ✓ 2 eggs
- ✓ 2 cups almond flour

Ingredients:

- ✓ 2 tablespoons coconut oil, spray
- ✓ 2 eggplants, peeled and thinly sliced Sunflower seeds and pepper

Directions:

- ❖ Preheat oven to 400 degrees F.
- ❖ Take a bowl and stir in sunflower seeds and black pepper.
- ❖ Take another bowl and beat the eggs until frothy.
- ❖ Dip the eggplant pieces into the eggs.

- ❖ Then coat them with the flour mixture.
- ❖ Add another layer of flour and eggs.
- ❖ Then, take a baking sheet and grease it with coconut oil on top.
- ❖ Bake for about 15 minutes. Serve and enjoy!

| **30) VERY WILD MUSHROOMS PILAF** | | |
|---|---|---|
| **Preparation Time**: 10 minutes | **Cooking Time**: 3 hours | **Servings**: 4 |

Ingredients:

- ✓ 1 cup wild rice
- ✓ 2 cloves minced garlic
- ✓ 6 chopped green onions

Ingredients:

- ✓ 2 tablespoons olive oil
- ✓ ½ pound baby Bella mushrooms
- ✓ 2 cups water

Directions:

- ❖ Add the rice, garlic, onion, oil, mushrooms and water to your Slow Cooker.
- ❖ Stir well until combined.
- ❖ Put the lid on and cook on LOW for 3 hours.
- ❖ Stir the pilaf and divide between serving plates. Enjoy!

---

| **31) SPORTS CARROTS FOR KIDS** | | |
|---|---|---|
| **Preparation Time**: 5 minutes | **Cooking Time**: 5 minutes | **Servings**: 4 |

Ingredients:

- ✓ 1 pound baby carrots
- ✓ 1 cup water

Ingredients:

- ✓ 1 tablespoon clarified ghee
- ✓ 1 tablespoon chopped fresh mint leaves
  Flavored sea vinegar, if needed

Directions:

- ❖ Place a steamer basket on top of your pot and add the carrots. Add the water.
- ❖ Close the lid and cook at HIGH pressure for 2 minutes. Make a quick release.
- ❖ Pass the carrots through a strainer and drain. Clean the insert.
- ❖ Return the insert to the pot and set the pot to Sauté mode. Add the clarified butter and let it melt.
- ❖ Add the mint and sauté for 30 seconds. Add the carrots to the insert and sauté well.
- ❖ Remove them and sprinkle some of the flavored vinegar on top. Enjoy!

| **32) GARDEN SALAD** | | |
|---|---|---|
| **Preparation Time**: 5 minutes | **Cooking Time**: 20 minutes | **Servings**: 6 |

Ingredients:

- ✓ 1 pound raw peanuts in shell
- ✓ 1 bay leaf
- ✓ 2 medium-sized tomatoes cut into pieces
- ✓ ½ cup diced green bell bell pepper
- ✓ ½ cup diced sweet onion

Ingredients:

- ✓ ¼ cup diced hot pepper
- ✓ ¼ cup diced celery
- ✓ 2 tablespoons olive oil
- ✓ ¾ teaspoon flavored vinegar
- ✓ ¼ teaspoon freshly ground black pepper

Directions:

- ❖ Boil your peanuts for 1 minute and rinse them.
- ❖ The skin will be soft, so discard it.
- ❖ Add 2 cups of water to the Instant Pot. Add the bay leaf and the peanuts.
- ❖ Close the lid and cook on high pressure for 20 minutes. Drain the water.
- ❖ Take a large bowl and add the peanuts, diced vegetables.
- ❖ Whisk the olive oil, lemon juice and pepper in another bowl.
- ❖ Pour the mixture over the salad and toss to combine. Enjoy!

## 33) BAKED SMOKED BROCCOLI WITH GARLIC

| Preparation Time: | Cooking Time: | Servings: |
|---|---|---|

**Ingredients:**

- ✓ cooking spray
- ✓ 1 tablespoon extra-virgin olive oil
- ✓ 3 cloves garlic, minced
- ✓ 1/2 teaspoon sea salt
- ✓ 1/4 teaspoon ground black pepper

**Ingredients:**

- ✓ ½ teaspoon cumin
- ✓ ½ teaspoon annatto seeds
- ✓ 3 1/2 cups sliced broccoli
- ✓ 1 lime, cut into wedges
- ✓ 1 tablespoon chopped fresh cilantro

**Directions:**

- ❖ Preheat oven to 450 degrees F. Line a baking sheet with aluminum foil and grease with olive oil.
- ❖ Mix the olive oil, garlic, cumin, annatto seeds, salt and pepper in a bowl.

- ❖ Add the cauliflower, carrots and broccoli and combine until well coated. Spread them in a single layer on the baking sheet.
- ❖ Add the lime wedges. Roast in the oven until the vegetables caramelize, about 25 minutes.
- ❖ Remove the lime wedges and add the cilantro.

## 34) ROASTED CAULIFLOWER AND LIMA BEANS

| Preparation Time: | Cooking Time: | Servings: |
|---|---|---|

**Ingredients:**

- ✓ cooking spray
- ✓ 1 tablespoon melted vegan butter/margarine
- ✓ 9 garlic cloves, minced
- ✓ 1/2 teaspoon sea salt
- ✓ 1/4 teaspoon ground black pepper

**Ingredients:**

- ✓ 1 1/2 cups sliced cauliflower
- ✓ 3 1/2 cups cherry tomatoes
- ✓ 1 (15-ounce) can lima beans, drained
- ✓ 1 lemon, cut into wedges

**Directions:**

- ❖ Preheat oven to 450 degrees F. Line a baking sheet with aluminum foil and grease with melted vegan butter or margarine.
- ❖ Mix the olive oil, garlic, salt and pepper in a bowl.

- ❖ Add the cauliflower, tomatoes and lima beans. Spread them in a single layer on the baking sheet.
- ❖ Add the lemon wedges.
- ❖ Roast in the oven until the vegetables caramelize, about 25 minutes. Remove the lemon wedges.

## 35) THAI SPICY ROASTED BLACK BEANS AND CHOY SUM

| Preparation Time: | Cooking Time: | Servings: |
|---|---|---|

**Ingredients:**

- ✓ 1 tablespoon sesame oil
- ✓ 3 garlic cloves, minced
- ✓ 1/2 teaspoon sea salt
- ✓ 1 tablespoon Thai chili paste
- ✓ 1/4 teaspoon ground black pepper

**Ingredients:**

- ✓ 3 1/2 cups Choy Sum, coarsely chopped
- ✓ 2 1/2 cups cherry tomatoes
- ✓ 1 (15-ounce) can black beans, drained
- ✓ 1 lime, cut into wedges
- ✓ 1 tablespoon chopped fresh cilantro

- ❖ Preheat oven to 450 degrees F. Line a baking sheet with aluminum foil and grease it with sesame oil.
- ❖ Mix the olive oil, garlic, salt, Thai chili paste and pepper in a bowl.
- ❖ Add the choy sum, tomatoes and black beans.

- ❖ Spread them in a single layer on the baking sheet.
- ❖ Add the lime wedges. Roast in the oven until the vegetables caramelize, about 25 minutes.
- ❖ Remove the lime wedges and add the cilantro.

## 36) PLAIN ROASTED BROCCOLI AND CAULIFLOWER

| Preparation Time: | Cooking Time: | Servings: |
|---|---|---|

**Ingredients:**

- ✓ 1 tablespoon extra virgin olive oil
- ✓ 3 cloves minced garlic
- ✓ 1/2 teaspoon sea salt
- ✓ 1/4 teaspoon ground black pepper

**Ingredients:**

- ✓ 3 1/2 cups broccoli
- ✓ 2 1/2 cups cauliflower
- ✓ 1 tablespoon chopped fresh thyme

**Directions:**

- ❖ Preheat oven to 450 degrees F.
- ❖ Line a baking sheet with aluminum foil and grease with olive oil. Mix the olive oil, garlic, salt and pepper in a bowl.

- ❖ Add the cauliflower and tomatoes and combine until well coated.
- ❖ Spread them out in a single layer on the baking sheet.
- ❖ Roast in the oven until the vegetables caramelize, about 25 minutes. Top with the thyme. Simple

## 37) ROASTED NAPA CABBAGE AND EXTRA TURNIPS

| Preparation Time: | Cooking Time: | Servings: |
|---|---|---|

**Ingredients:**

- ✓ cooking spray
- ✓ 1 tablespoon extra virgin olive oil
- ✓ 1/2 teaspoon sea salt

**Ingredients:**

- ✓ 1/4 teaspoon ground black pepper
- ✓ 1/2 medium Napa cabbage, thinly sliced
- ✓ 1 medium turnip, thinly sliced

**Directions:**

- ❖ Preheat oven to 450 degrees F.
- ❖ Line a baking sheet with aluminum foil and grease with olive oil.
- ❖ Mix the extra ingredients together well.

- ❖ Add the main ingredients and combine until well coated.
- ❖ Spread in a single layer on the baking sheet.
- ❖ Roast in oven until vegetables become caramelized, about 25 minutes.

## 38) SIMPLE ROASTED CABBAGE WITH ARTICHOKE HEART AND EXTRA CHOY SUM

| Preparation Time: | Cooking Time: | Servings: |
|---|---|---|

**Ingredients:**

- ✓ 1 tablespoon extra virgin olive oil
- ✓ 1/2 teaspoon sea salt
- ✓ 1/4 teaspoon ground black pepper Main ingredients

**Ingredients:**

- ✓ 1 bunch cabbage, rinsed and drained
- ✓ 1 cup canned artichoke hearts
- ✓ 1/2 medium-flowered Chinese cabbage (choy sum), roughly chopped

**Directions:**

- ❖ Preheat oven to 450 degrees F. Line a baking sheet with aluminum foil and grease with olive oil.
- ❖ Mix the extra ingredients together well.

- ❖ Add the main ingredients and combine until well coated.
- ❖ Spread in a single layer on the baking sheet.
- ❖ Roast in oven until vegetables become caramelized, about 25 minutes.

## 39) ROASTED CABBAGE AND BOK CHOY EXTRA

| Preparation Time: | Cooking Time: | Servings: |
|---|---|---|

**Ingredients:**

- ✓ 1 tablespoon extra virgin olive oil
- ✓ 1/2 teaspoon sea salt
- ✓ 1/4 teaspoon ground black pepper

**Directions:**

- ❖ Preheat oven to 450 degrees F.
- ❖ Line a baking sheet with aluminum foil and grease with olive oil.
- ❖ Mix the extra ingredients together well.

**Ingredients:**

- ✓ 1 bunch kale, rinsed and drained
- ✓ 1 bunch bok choy, rinsed, drained and coarsely chopped

- ❖ Add the main ingredients and combine until well coated.
- ❖ Spread in a single layer on the baking sheet.
- ❖ Roast in oven until vegetables become caramelized, about 25 minutes.

---

## 40) ROASTED SOY BEANS AND WINTER SQUASH

| Preparation Time: | Cooking Time: | Servings: |
|---|---|---|

**Ingredients:**

- ✓ 2 (15-ounce) cans of soybeans, rinsed and drained
- ✓ 1/2 winter squash - peeled, seeded and cut into 1-inch pieces 1 red onion, diced
- ✓ 1 sweet potato, peeled and cut into 1-inch cubes
- ✓ 2 large carrots, cut into 1-inch pieces
- ✓ 3 medium potatoes
- ✓ 4 tablespoons extra virgin olive oil Ingredients for seasoning

**Ingredients:**

- ✓ 1 teaspoon salt
- ✓ 1/2 teaspoon ground black pepper
- ✓ 1 teaspoon onion powder
- ✓ 1 teaspoon dried basil
- ✓ 1 teaspoon Italian seasoning Ingredients for garnishes
- ✓ 2 green onions, chopped (optional)

**Directions:**

- ❖ Preheat oven to 350 degrees F.
- ❖ Grease baking sheet. Combine beans, squash, onion, sweet potato, carrots and russet potatoes on prepared baking sheet. Drizzle with oil and toss to coat.
- ❖ Combine the dressing ingredients in a bowl, spread over the vegetables on the baking sheet and toss to coat with the dressing.

- ❖ Bake in the oven for 25 minutes. Stir often until the vegetables are soft and lightly browned and the beans are crisp, about 20-25 minutes more.
- ❖ Season with more salt and black pepper to taste, add green onion before serving.

## 41) ROASTED CHAMPIGNON MUSHROOMS AND PUMPKIN

| Preparation Time: | Cooking Time: | Servings: |
|---|---|---|

**Ingredients:**

- ✓ 2 (15-ounce) cans button mushrooms, rinsed and drained
- ✓ 1/2 summer squash - peeled, seeded and cut into 1-inch pieces
- ✓ 1 red onion, diced
- ✓ 2 large turnips, cut into 1-inch pieces
- ✓ 2 large parsnips, cut into 1-inch pieces
- ✓ 3 medium potatoes, cut into 1-inch pieces
- ✓ 3 tablespoons butter Ingredients for seasoning

**Ingredients:**

- ✓ 1 teaspoon salt
- ✓ 1/2 teaspoon ground black pepper
- ✓ 1 teaspoon onion powder
- ✓ 2 teaspoons garlic powder
- ✓ 1 teaspoon Herbes de Provence Ingredients for garnishes
- ✓ 2 sprigs thyme, chopped (optional)

**Directions:**

- ❖ Preheat oven to 350 degrees F.
- ❖ Grease baking dish. Combine main ingredients on prepared baking sheet.
- ❖ Drizzle with melted butter or margarine and toss to coat. Combine the topping ingredients in a bowl, spread over the vegetables on the baking sheet and stir to coat with the toppings.

- ❖ Bake for 25 minutes. Stir often until the vegetables are soft and lightly browned and the chickpeas are crisp, about another 20-25 minutes.
- ❖ Season with more salt and black pepper to taste, add thyme before serving.

---

## 42) ROASTED TOMATOES RUTABAGA AND KOHLRABI

| Preparation Time: | Cooking Time: | Servings: |
|---|---|---|

**Ingredients:**

- ✓ 3 large tomatoes, cut into 1-inch pieces
- ✓ 3 red onion, diced
- ✓ 1 rutabaga, peeled and cut into 1-inch cubes
- ✓ 2 large carrots, cut into 1-inch pieces
- ✓ 3 medium kohlrabi, cut into 1-inch pieces
- ✓ 3 tablespoons extra virgin olive oil Ingredients for seasoning
- ✓ 1 teaspoon salt

**Ingredients:**

- ✓ 1/2 teaspoon ground black pepper
- ✓ 1 teaspoon onion powder
- ✓ 2 teaspoons garlic powder
- ✓ 1 teaspoon Spanish paprika
- ✓ 1 teaspoon cumin Ingredients for garnishes
- ✓ 2 sprigs parsley, chopped (optional)

**Directions:**

- ❖ Preheat oven to 350 degrees F. Grease baking sheet. Combine main ingredients on prepared baking sheet.
- ❖ Drizzle with oil and toss to coat. Combine dressing ingredients in a bowl, spread over vegetables on baking sheet and toss to coat with dressing.

- ❖ Bake in the oven for 25 minutes. Stir often until vegetables are soft, about 20-25 minutes more.
- ❖ Season with more salt and black pepper to taste, add parsley before serving.

## 43) BRUSSELS SPROUTS AND ROASTED BROCCOLI

| Preparation Time: | Cooking Time: | Servings: |
|---|---|---|

**Ingredients:**

- ✓ 1 large broccoli, sliced
- ✓ 1 cup bean sprouts
- ✓ 1 red onion, diced
- ✓ 3 large kohlrabi, cut into 1-inch pieces
- ✓ 2 large carrots, cut into 1-inch pieces
- ✓ 3 medium potatoes, cut into 1-inch pieces
- ✓ 3 tablespoons extra virgin olive oil Ingredients for dressing

**Ingredients:**

- ✓ 1 teaspoon salt
- ✓ 1/2 teaspoon ground black pepper
- ✓ 1 teaspoon onion powder
- ✓ 2 teaspoons garlic powder
- ✓ 1 teaspoon ground fennel seeds
- ✓ 1 teaspoon dried rubbed sage Ingredients for garnishes
- ✓ 2 green onions, chopped (optional)

**Directions:**

- ❖ Preheat oven to 350 degrees F. Grease baking sheet.
- ❖ Combine main ingredients on prepared baking sheet. Drizzle with oil and toss to coat.
- ❖ Combine dressing ingredients in a bowl, spread over vegetables on baking sheet and toss to coat with dressing. Bake in the oven for 25 minutes.

- ❖ Stir often until the vegetables are soft and lightly browned and the chickpeas are crisp, about 20-25 more minutes.
- ❖ Season with more salt and black pepper to taste, add green onion before serving.

## 44) ROASTED BROCCOLI, SWEET POTATOES AND BEAN SPROUTS

| Preparation Time: | Cooking Time: | Servings: |
|---|---|---|

**Ingredients:**

- ✓ 1 large broccoli, sliced
- ✓ 1 cup bean sprouts
- ✓ 1 yellow onion, diced
- ✓ 1 sweet potato, peeled and cut into 1-inch cubes
- ✓ 2 large carrots, cut into 1-inch pieces
- ✓ 3 medium potatoes, cut into 1-inch pieces
- ✓ 3 tablespoons canola oil Ingredients for the dressing

**Ingredients:**

- ✓ 1 teaspoon salt
- ✓ 1/2 teaspoon ground black pepper
- ✓ 1 teaspoon onion powder
- ✓ 2 teaspoons garlic powder
- ✓ ½ cup grated gouda cheese
- ✓ ¼ cup Parmesan cheese
- ✓ 2 green onions, chopped (optional)

**Directions:**

- ❖ Preheat oven to 350 degrees F. Grease baking dish. Combine main ingredients on prepared baking sheet. Drizzle with oil and toss to coat.
- ❖ Combine dressing ingredients in a bowl, spread over vegetables on baking sheet and toss to coat with dressing. Bake in the oven for 25 minutes.

- ❖ Stir often until the vegetables are soft and lightly browned and the chickpeas are crisp, about another 20-25 minutes.
- ❖ Season with more salt and black pepper to taste, add green onion before serving.

## 45) SWEET POTATOES AND ROASTED RED BEETS

| Preparation Time: | Cooking Time: | Servings: |
|---|---|---|

**Ingredients:**

- ✓ 1 ½ cups Brussels sprouts, cut
- ✓ 1 cup large sweet potatoes, chopped
- ✓ 1 cup large carrots, chopped
- ✓ 1 ½ cups broccoli florets

**Ingredients:**

- ✓ 1 cup diced red beets
- ✓ 1/2 cup yellow onion, chopped
- ✓ 2 tablespoons sesame seed oil salt and ground black pepper to taste

**Directions:**

- ❖ Preheat the oven to 425 degrees F (220 degrees C).
- ❖ Set the rack to the second lowest level of the oven. Pour lightly salted water into a bowl.
- ❖ Soak Brussels sprouts in salted water for 15 minutes and drain.

- ❖ Place the rest of the ingredients in a bowl.
- ❖ Spread the vegetables in a single layer on a baking sheet.
- ❖ Roast in the oven until the vegetables begin to brown and cook, about 45 minutes.

## 46) BEETS AND BROCCOLI FLORETS BAKED SICHUAN STYLE

| Preparation Time: | Cooking Time: | Servings: |
|---|---|---|

**Ingredients:**

- ✓ 1 ½ cups Brussels sprouts, chopped
- ✓ 1 cup broccoli florets
- ✓ 1 cup Choggia beets, chopped
- ✓ 1 ½ cups cauliflower florets

**Ingredients:**

- ✓ 1 cup button mushrooms, sliced
- ✓ 1/2 cup chopped red onion
- ✓ 2 tablespoons sesame oil
- ✓ ½ teaspoon Sichuan pepper salt ground black pepper to taste

**Directions:**

- ❖ Preheat the oven to 425 degrees F (220 degrees C).
- ❖ Set the rack to the second lowest level of the oven. Pour lightly salted water into a bowl.

- ❖ Soak Brussels sprouts in salted water for 15 minutes and drain. Place the rest of the ingredients in a bowl.
- ❖ Spread the vegetables in a single layer on a baking sheet.
- ❖ Roast in the oven until the vegetables begin to brown and cook, about 45 minutes.

## 47) BAKED ENOKI AND MINI CABBAGE

| Preparation Time: | Cooking Time: | Servings: |
|---|---|---|

**Ingredients:**

- ✓ 1 ½ cups mini cabbage, chopped
- ✓ 1 cup broccoli florets
- ✓ 1 cup enoki mushrooms, sliced
- ✓ 1 ½ cups cauliflower florets

**Ingredients:**

- ✓ 1 cup oyster mushrooms
- ✓ 1/2 cup chopped red onion
- ✓ 2 tablespoons olive oil salt and ground black pepper to taste

**Directions:**

- ❖ Preheat the oven to 425 degrees F (220 degrees C).
- ❖ Set the rack to the second lowest level of the oven.
- ❖ Pour lightly salted water into a bowl. Soak Brussels sprouts in salted water for 15 minutes and drain.

- ❖ Place the rest of the ingredients in a bowl.
- ❖ Spread the vegetables in a single layer on a baking sheet.
- ❖ Roast in the oven until the vegetables begin to brown and cook, about 45 minutes.

## 48) TRIPLE ROASTED MUSHROOMS

| Preparation Time: | Cooking Time: | Servings: |
|---|---|---|

**Ingredients:**

- ✓ 2 cups spinach, rinsed
- ✓ 1 cup oyster mushrooms
- ✓ 1 cup button mushrooms, sliced
- ✓ 1 ½ cups enoki mushrooms

**Ingredients:**

- ✓ 1/2 cup chopped red onion
- ✓ 2 tablespoons extra virgin olive oil salt and ground black pepper to taste
- ✓ 1/4 cup ricotta cheese

**Directions:**

- ❖ Preheat the oven to 425 degrees F (220 degrees C).
- ❖ Set the rack to the second lowest level of the oven. Pour lightly salted water into a bowl.
- ❖ Soak spinach in salted water for 15 minutes and drain.

- ❖ Place the rest of the ingredients in a bowl.
- ❖ Spread the vegetables in a single layer on a baking sheet. Roast in the oven until the vegetables begin to brown and cook, about 45 minutes.

## 49) MINI ROASTED CABBAGE AND SWEET POTATOES

| Preparation Time: | Cooking Time: | Servings: |
|---|---|---|

**Ingredients:**

- ✓ 1 ½ cups mini cabbage, cut
- ✓ 1 cup large pieces of potatoes
- ✓ 1 cup large pieces of rainbow carrots
- ✓ 1 ½ cup pieces of potatoes

**Ingredients:**

- ✓ 1 cup parsnips
- ✓ 1/2 cup pieces of red onion
- ✓ 2 tablespoons extra virgin olive oil Sea salt Rainbow pepper to taste
- ✓ 1/4 cup cottage cheese

**Directions:**

- ❖ Preheat the oven to 425 degrees F (220 degrees C).
- ❖ Set the rack to the second lowest level of the oven. Pour lightly salted water into a bowl.
- ❖ Soak mini cabbage in salted water for 15 minutes and drain.

- ❖ Place the rest of the ingredients in a bowl. Spread the vegetables in a single layer on a baking sheet.
- ❖ Roast in the oven until the vegetables begin to brown and cook, about 45 minutes.

# Chapter 3. DINNER

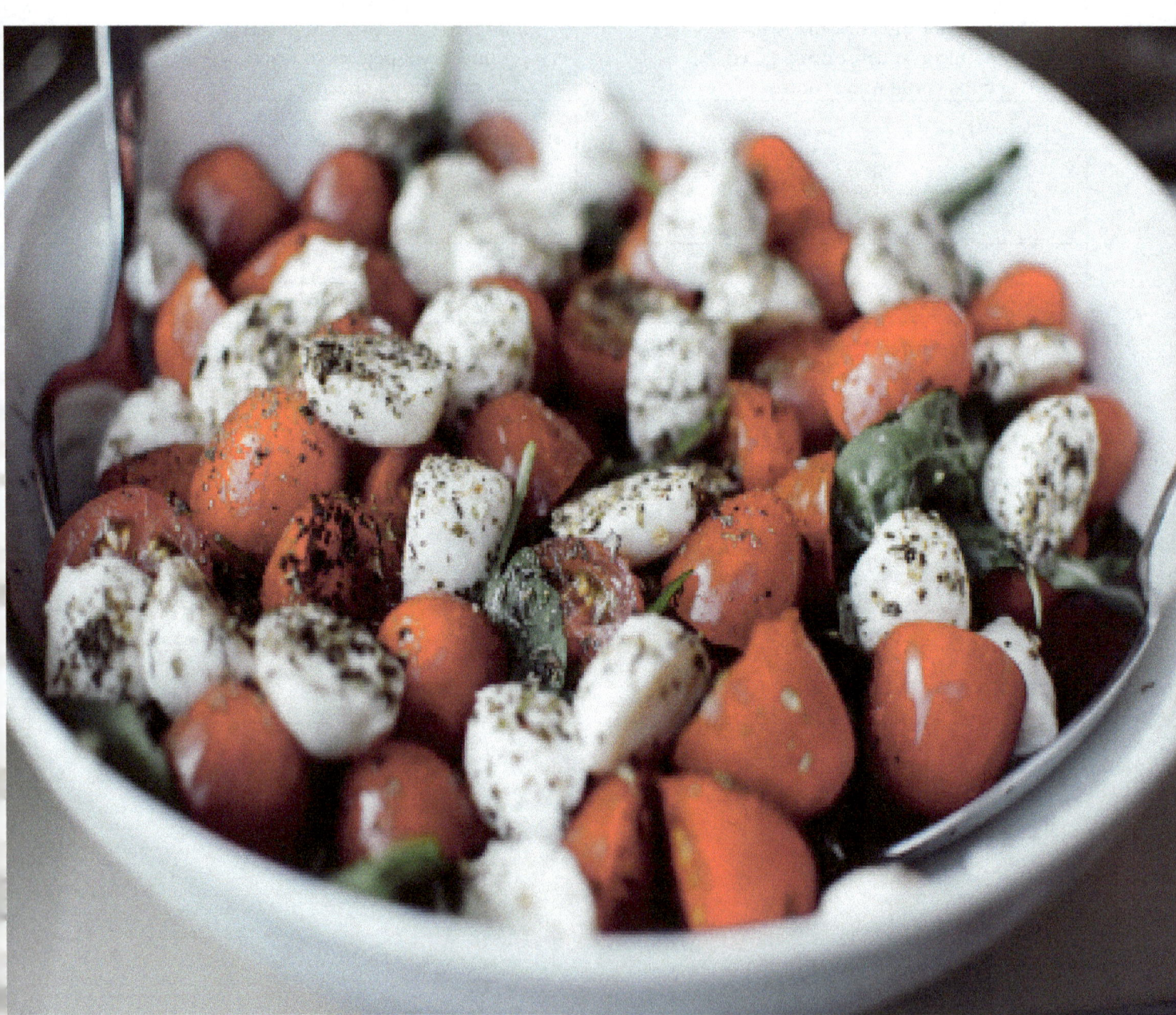

## 50) CURRIED BEEF MEATBALLS

| **Preparation Time**: 20 minutes | **Cooking Time:** 22 minutes | **Servings: 6** |
| --- | --- | --- |

Ingredients:

- ✓ For the meatballs:
- ✓ 1 pound lean ground beef
- ✓ 2 organic eggs, bea10
- ✓ 3 tablespoons red onion, chopped
- ✓ ¼ cup fresh basil leaves, chopped
- ✓ 1 (1-inch) piece fresh ginger, finely chopped
- ✓ 4 cloves garlic, finely chopped
- ✓ 3 Thai bird's eye chilies, chopped
- ✓ 1 tablespoon coconut sugar
- ✓ 1 tablespoon red curry paste - Salt, to taste –
- ✓ 1 tablespoon fish sauce

Ingredients:

- ✓ 2 tablespoons coconut oil

  For Curry:
- ✓ 1 red onion, chopped - Salt, to taste
- ✓ 4 garlic cloves, chopped
- ✓ 1 piece fresh ginger (1 inch), chopped
- ✓ 2 Thai chilies, chopped
- ✓ 2 tablespoons red curry paste
- ✓ 1 coconut milk (14 ounces) - Salt and freshly ground black pepper, to taste
- ✓ Lime wedge, to serve

Directions:

- ❖ For meatballs in a large bowl, add all ingredients except oil and mix until well combined. Make small balls from the mixture. In a large skillet, melt the coconut oil over medium heat. Add the patties and cook for about 3-5 minutes or until golden brown on all sides.

- ❖ Transfer the meatballs to a bowl. In the same skillet, add the onion and a pinch of salt and sauté for about 5 minutes. Add the garlic, ginger and chilies and sauté for about 1 minute. Add the curry paste and stir-fry for about 1 minute.
- ❖ Add the coconut milk and meatballs and bring to a boil over low heat. Reduce heat to low and simmer, covered for about 10 minutes. Serve with the lime wedge dressing.

## 51) GRILLED STEAK WITH COCONUT

| **Preparation Time**: 15 minutes | **Cooking Time:** 8-9 minutes | **Servings: 4** |
| --- | --- | --- |

Ingredients:

- ✓ 2 teaspoons fresh ginger, finely grated
- ✓ 2 teaspoons fresh lime zest, finely grated
- ✓ ¼ cup coconut sugar
- ✓ 2 teaspoons fish sauce

Ingredients:

- ✓ 2 tablespoons fresh lime juice
- ✓ ½ cup coconut milk
- ✓ 1 pound beef skirt steak, trimmed and cut into 4-inch slices lengthwise
- ✓ Salt, to taste

Directions:

- ❖ In a resealable bag, mix all ingredients except steak and salt. Add the steak and coat generously with the marinade. Seal the bag and refrigerate to marinate for about 4-12 hours. Preheat grill to high heat. Grease the grill grate. Remove the steak from the refrigerator and discard the marinade.

- ❖ Using a paper towel, pat the steak dry and sprinkle with salt evenly. Cook the steak for about 3 1/2 minutes. Turn the middle side out and cook for about 2½ to 5 minutes or until desired doneness.
- ❖ Remove from grill pan and hold side for about 5 minutes before slicing. Using a clear, crisp knife, cut into desired slices and serve.

## 52) LAMB WITH PRUNES

| **Preparation Time**: 15 minutes | **Cooking Time:** a couple of hours and 40 minutes | **Servings: 4-6** |
|---|---|---|

Ingredients:

- ✓ 3 tablespoons coconut oil
- ✓ 2 onions, finely chopped
- ✓ 1 (1-inch) piece of fresh ginger, chopped
- ✓ 3 garlic cloves, chopped
- ✓ ½ teaspoon turmeric powder
- ✓ 2 ½ lbs. of lamb shoulder, trimmed and cut into 3-inch cubes

Ingredients:

- ✓ Salt and freshly ground black pepper, to taste
- ✓ ½ teaspoon saffron threads, crumbled
- ✓ 1 cinnamon stick
- ✓ 3 cups water
- ✓ 1 cup runes, pitted and halved

Directions:

- ❖ In a large skillet, melt the coconut oil over medium heat. Add the onions, ginger, garlic cloves and turmeric and sauté for about 3-5 minutes. Sprinkle the lamb evenly with salt and black pepper. In the skillet, add the lamb and saffron threads and cook for about 4-5 minutes.

- ❖ Add the cinnamon stick and water and produce to a boil over high heat. Reduce the heat to low and simmer, covered for about 1½-120 minutes or until the lamb has reached the desired temperature.
- ❖ Add the plums and simmer for about 20½ hours. Remove the cinnamon stick and serve hot.

## 53) GROUND LAMB WITH PEAS

| **Preparation Time**: 15 minutes | **Cooking Time:** 55 minutes | **Servings: 4** |
|---|---|---|

Ingredients:

- ✓ 1 tablespoon coconut oil
- ✓ 3 dried red chilies
- ✓ 1 cinnamon stick (2 inches)
- ✓ 3 green cardamom pods
- ✓ ½ teaspoon cumin seeds
- ✓ 1 medium red onion, chopped
- ✓ 1 piece fresh ginger (¾ inch), chopped
- ✓ 4 cloves garlic, minced
- ✓ 1½ teaspoons ground coriander
- ✓ ½ teaspoon garam masala
- ✓ ½ teaspoon ground cumin

Ingredients:

- ✓ ½ teaspoon ground turmeric
- ✓ ¼ teaspoon ground nutmeg
- ✓ 2 bay leaves
- ✓ 1 pound ground lean lamb
- ✓ ½ cup Roma tomatoes, chopped
- ✓ 1-1½ cup water
- ✓ 1 cup fresh green peas, shelled
- ✓ 2 tablespoons plain Greek yogurt, whipped
- ✓ ¼ cup fresh cilantro, chopped
- ✓ Salt and freshly ground black pepper, to taste

Directions:

- ❖ In a Dutch oven, melt the coconut oil over medium-high heat. Add the red chiles, cinnamon stick, cardamom pods and cumin seeds and sauté for about thirty seconds. Add the onion and sauté for about 3-4 minutes.

- ❖ Add the ginger, garlic cloves and spices and sauté for about thirty seconds. Add the lamb and cook about 5 minutes. Add the tomatoes and cook about 10 minutes. Add the water and green peas and cook covered for about 25-30 minutes.
- ❖ Add the yogurt, cilantro, salt and black pepper and cook for about 4-5 minutes. Serve hot.

## 54) ROAST LAMB CHOPS

| **Preparation Time**: 15 minutes | **Cooking Time:** half an hour | **Servings: 4** |
|---|---|---|

Ingredients:

For the lamb marinade:
- ✓ 4 cloves garlic, chopped
- ✓ 1 (2 inch) piece fresh ginger, chopped
- ✓ 2 green chiles, seeded and chopped
- ✓ 1 teaspoon fresh lime zest
- ✓ 2 teaspoons garam masala
- ✓ 1 teaspoon ground coriander
- ✓ 1 teaspoon ground cumin
- ✓ ½ teaspoon ground cinnamon
- ✓ 1 teaspoon coconut oil, melted
- ✓ 2 tablespoons fresh lime juice
- ✓ 6-7 tablespoons plain Greek yogurt
- ✓ 1 (8-bone) rack of lamb, chopped

Ingredients:
- ✓ 2 onions, sliced

For Relish:
- ✓ ½ of garlic, chopped
- ✓ 1 (1-inch) piece of fresh ginger, chopped
- ✓ ¼ cup fresh cilantro, chopped
- ✓ ¼ cup fresh mint, chopped
- ✓ 1 green chile, seeded and chopped
- ✓ 1 teaspoon fresh lime zest
- ✓ 1 teaspoon organic honey
- ✓ 2 tablespoons fresh apple juice
- ✓ 2 tablespoons fresh lime juice

❖ For the chops in a very mixer, add all ingredients except the yogurt, chops and onions and pulse until smooth. Transfer the mixture to a large bowl with the yogurt and stir to combine well. Add the chops and coat generously with the mixture. Refrigerate to marinate for about twenty-four hours.

❖ Preheat oven to 375 degrees F. Line baking sheet with aluminum foil. Place the onion wedges in the bottom of the prepared baking dish. Arrange rack of lamb on top of onion wedges. Roast about half an hour. Meanwhile for relish in blender, add all ingredients and pulse until smooth. Serve the chops and onions along with the relish.

## 55) MEATBALLS BAKED WITH SHALLOTS

| **Preparation Time**: 20 minutes | **Cooking Time:** 35 minutes | **Servings: 4-6** |
|---|---|---|

Ingredients:

For the patties:
- ✓ 1 lemongrass stalk, outer peel peeled and chopped
- ✓ 1 (1½-inch) piece fresh ginger, sliced –
- ✓ 3 garlic cloves, chopped
- ✓ 1 cup fresh cilantro leaves, coarsely chopped
- ✓ ½ cup fresh basil leaves, coarsely chopped
- ✓ 2 tablespoons plus 1 teaspoon fish sauce
- ✓ 2 tablespoons water
- ✓ 2 tablespoons fresh lime juice

Ingredients:
- ✓ ½ pound lean ground pork
- ✓ 1 pound lean ground lamb
- ✓ 1 carrot, peeled and grated
- ✓ 1 organic egg, bea10
- ✓ For the scallions: -
- ✓ 16 scallion stalks, chopped
- ✓ 2 tablespoons coconut oil, melted - Salt, to taste
- ✓ ½ cup water

Directions:

❖ Preheat oven to 375 degrees F. Grease a baking sheet. In a blender, add the lemongrass, ginger, garlic, fresh herbs, fish sauce, water and lime juice and blend until finely chopped.

❖ Transfer the amalgam to a bowl with the remaining ingredients and mix until well combined. Make 1-inch balls from the mixture.

❖ Arrange the balls in the prepared baking dish in a single layer. In another rimmed baking dish, arrange shallot stalks in a single layer. Drizzle with coconut oil and sprinkle with salt. Pour the water into the baking dish and cover 1 tightly with aluminum foil.

❖ Cook the shallots for about half an hour.. Bake the meatballs for about 30-35 minutes. Pork with peppers This stir-fry doesn't just taste wonderful, it's also full of nutritious benefits.

## 56) PORK CHILI

| **Preparation Time**: 15 minutes | **Cooking Time**: 60 minutes | **Servings: 8** |
|---|---|---|

Ingredients:

- ✓ 2 tbsp. organic extra virgin olive oil
- ✓ 2 lbs. ground pork
- ✓ 1 medium red bell pepper, seeded and chopped
- ✓ 1 medium onion, chopped
- ✓ 5 cloves of garlic, finely chopped
- ✓ 1 part (2 in.) of chili pepper, ground
- ✓ 1 tablespoon ground cumin
- ✓ 1 teaspoon ground turmeric

Ingredients:

- ✓ 3 tablespoons chili powder
- ✓ ½ teaspoon chipotle chili powder - Salt and freshly ground black pepper, to taste
- ✓ 1 cup chicken broth
- ✓ 1 (28-ounce) can fire-roasted tomatoes, crushed
- ✓ 2 medium bokchoy heads, sliced
- ✓ 1 avocado, peeled, pitted and chopped

Directions:

❖ In a large skillet, heat oil over medium heat. Add the pork and sauté for about 5 minutes. Add the bell bell pepper, onion, garlic, chili and spices and sauté for about 5 minutes. Add the broth and tomatoes and bring to a boil.

❖

❖ Add the bokchoy and cook, covered for about twenty minutes. Uncover and cook for about 20 ½ hours. Serve warm while using an avocado garnish.

## 57) PORK MEATBALLS AND BAKED MUSHROOMS

| **Preparation Time**: 15 minutes | **Cooking Time**: 15 minutes | **Servings: 6** |
|---|---|---|

Ingredients:

- ✓ 1 pound lean pork
- ✓ 1 egg white,
- ✓ 4 fresh shiitake mushrooms, cut and chopped
- ✓ 1 tablespoon fresh parsley, chopped
- ✓ 1 tablespoon fresh basil leaves, chopped

Ingredients:

- ✓ 1 tablespoon fresh mint leaves, chopped
- ✓ 2 teaspoons fresh lemon zest, finely grated
- ✓ 1½ teaspoons fresh ginger, finely grated
- ✓ Salt and freshly ground black pepper, to taste

Directions:

❖ Preheat the oven to 425 degrees F. Place the rack in the center of the oven. Line a baking sheet with parchment paper. In a sizable bowl, add all ingredients and mix until well combined.

❖ Make small balls of equal size from the mixture. Arrange the balls on the prepared baking sheet in a single layer. Bake for about 12 quarters of an hour or until cooked through.

## 58) BEEF WITH CITRUS FRUITS AND BOK CHOY

| **Preparation Time**: 15 minutes | **Cooking Time:** 11 minutes | **Servings: 4** |
|---|---|---|

Ingredients:

For the marinade:
- ✓ 2 cloves minced garlic
- ✓ 1 (1-inch) piece fresh ginger, grated
- ✓ 1/3 cup fresh orange juice
- ✓ ½ cup coconut aminos
- ✓ 2 teaspoons fish sauce
- ✓ 2 teaspoons Sriracha
- ✓ 1¼ pounds sirloin steak, thinly sliced and cut

Ingredients:

For the vegetables:
- ✓ 2 tablespoons coconut oil, divided
- ✓ 3-4 wide strips of fresh orange zest
- ✓ 1 jalapeño bell pepper, thinly sliced
- ✓ ½ pound green beans, cut and halved crosswise
- ✓ 1 tablespoon arrowroot powder
- ✓ ½ pound bokchoy, chopped
- ✓ 2 teaspoons sesame seeds

Directions:

❖ For the marinade in a large bowl, mix together garlic, ginger, orange juice, coconut aminos, fish sauce and Sriracha. Add beef and coat generously with marinade. Refrigerate to marinate for about a couple of hours. In a substantial skillet, heat oil over medium-high heat. Add the orange zest and sauté about 2 minutes.

❖ Remove the beef from the bowl, reserving the marinade. In the skillet, add the beef and increase the heat to high.

❖ Sauté for about 2-3 minutes or until golden brown. Using a slotted spoon, transfer the beef and orange strips to a bowl. Using a paper towel, pat the pan dry. In a similar skillet, heat the remaining oil over medium-high heat.

❖ Add the jalapeño bell pepper and green beans and sauté for about 3-4 minutes. Meanwhile, add the arrowroot powder to the reserved marinade and stir to combine. In the skillet, add the marinade mixture, beef and bokchoy and cook for about 1-2 minutes. Serve hot with sesame seed garnish.

## 59) GROUND BEEF WITH CABBAGE

| **Preparation Time**: 10 minutes | **Cooking Time:** 15 minutes | **Servings: 6** |
|---|---|---|

Ingredients:

- ✓ 1 tablespoon olive oil
- ✓ 1 onion, thinly sliced
- ✓ 2 teaspoons fresh ginger, chopped
- ✓ 4 cloves garlic, chopped
- ✓ 1 pound lean ground beef

Ingredients:

- ✓ 1½ tablespoons fish sauce
- ✓ 2 tablespoons fresh lime juice
- ✓ 1 small head of purple cabbage, shredded
- ✓ 2 tablespoons peanut butter
- ✓ ½ cup fresh cilantro, chopped

Directions:

❖ In a large skillet, heat the oil over medium heat. Add the onion, ginger and garlic and sauté for about 4-5 minutes. Add the beef and cook for about 7-8 minutes, breaking it up with a spoon.

❖ Drain off the extra liquid in the skillet. Stir in the fish sauce and lime juice and cook for about 1 minute. Add the cabbage and cook about 4-5 minutes or until desired doneness. Add the peanut butter and cilantro and cook for about 1 minute. Serve hot.

## 60) BEEF CHILI WITH VEGETABLES

| **Preparation Time**: 15 minutes | **Cooking Time**: 1 hour | **Servings**: 6-8 |
| --- | --- | --- |

Ingredients:

- ✓ 2 lbs. lean ground beef
- ✓ - ½ head of cauliflower, cut into large pieces
- ✓ - 1 onion, chopped
- ✓ - 6 cloves of garlic, chopped
- ✓ - 2 cups of pumpkin puree
- ✓ - 1 tsp. dried oregano, crushed
- ✓ - 1 tsp. dried thyme, crushed
- ✓ - 1 teaspoon ground cumin
- ✓ - 1 teaspoon ground turmeric

Ingredients:

- ✓ - 1-2 teaspoons chili powder
- ✓ - 1 teaspoon paprika
- ✓ - 1 teaspoon cayenne pepper
- ✓ - ¼ teaspoon red pepper flakes, crushed - Salt and freshly ground black pepper, to taste
- ✓ - 1 (26-ounce) can tomatoes, drained
- ✓ - ½ cup water
- ✓ - 1 cup meat stock

Directions:

- ❖ Heat a substantial skillet over medium-high heat. Add the beef and sauté for about 5 minutes. Add the cauliflower, onion and garlic and sauté for about 5 minutes.

- ❖ Add the spices and herbs and stir to mix well. Reduce heat to low and simmer, covered for about 30-45 minutes. Serve hot.

## 61) BEEF MEATBALLS IN TOMATO SAUCE

| **Preparation Time**: 20 minutes | **Cooking Time**: 37 minutes | **Servings**: 4 |
| --- | --- | --- |

Ingredients:

For the meatballs:
- ✓ - 1 pound lean ground beef
- ✓ - 1 organic egg
- ✓ - 1 tablespoon fresh ginger, chopped
- ✓ - 1 garlic oil, chopped
- ✓ - 2 tablespoons fresh cilantro, finely chopped
- ✓ - 2 tablespoons tomato paste
- ✓ - 1/3 cup almond flour
- ✓ - 1 tablespoon ground cumin –
- ✓ Pinch of ground cinnamon - Salt and freshly ground black pepper, to taste
- ✓ - ¼ cup coconut oil

Ingredients:

For the tomato sauce:
- ✓ - 2 tablespoons coconut oil
- ✓ - ½ small onion, chopped
- ✓ - 2 cloves garlic, chopped
- ✓ - 1 teaspoon fresh lemon zest, finely grated
- ✓ - 2 cups tomatoes, finely chopped
- ✓ - Pinch of ground cinnamon
- ✓ - 1 teaspoon red pepper flakes, crushed
- ✓ - ¾ cup chicken broth - Salt and freshly ground black pepper, to taste
- ✓ - ¼ cup fresh parsley, chopped

Directions:

- ❖ For the meatballs, in a large bowl, add all ingredients except oil and mix until well combined. Make balls about 1 inch from the mixture. In a substantial skillet, melt the coconut oil over medium heat. Add the patties and cook for about 3-5 minutes or until golden brown on all sides.

- ❖ Transfer the meatballs to a bowl. For the sauce in a large skillet, melt the coconut oil over medium heat. Add the onion and garlic and sauté about 4 minutes. Add the lemon zest and sauté about 1 minute.
- ❖ Add the tomatoes, cinnamon, red pepper flakes and broth and simmer about 7 minutes. Add the salt, black pepper and meatballs and reduce the heat to medium-low. Simmer for about twenty minutes. Serve hot with all the parsley garnishes.

## 62) SPICY LAMB CURRY

| **Preparation Time**: 15 minutes | **Cooking Time**: 2 quarter hours | **Servings: 6-8** |
| --- | --- | --- |

Ingredients:

For the spice blend:
- ✓ - 4 teaspoons ground coriander
- ✓ - 4 teaspoons ground cumin
- ✓ - ¾ teaspoon ground ginger
- ✓ - 2 teaspoons ground cinnamon
- ✓ - ½ teaspoon ground cloves
- ✓ - ½ teaspoon ground cardamom
- ✓ - 2 tablespoons sweet paprika
- ✓ - ½ teaspoon cayenne pepper
- ✓ - 2 teaspoons chili powder

Ingredients:

- ✓ - 2 teaspoons salt

For the Curry:
- ✓ - 1 tablespoon coconut oil
- ✓ - 2 pounds boneless lamb, trimmed and cut into 1-inch cubes - Salt and freshly ground black pepper, to taste
- ✓ - 2 cups onions, chopped
- ✓ - 1¼ cups water
- ✓ - 1 cup coconut milk

Directions:

❖ For the spice mixture in a bowl, mix together all the spices. Keep aside. Season lamb with salt and black pepper. In a large Dutch oven, heat oil over medium-high heat. Add the lamb and sauté for about 5 minutes.

❖ Add the onion and cook about 4-5 minutes. Add the spice mixture and cook for about 1 minute. Add the water and coconut milk and bring to a boil over high heat. Reduce heat to low and simmer, covered for about 1-120 minutes or until desired doneness of lamb. Uncover and simmer for about 3-4 minutes. Serve hot.

## 63) GROUND LAMB WITH HARISSA

| **Preparation Time**: 15 minutes | **Cooking Time**: 1 hour 11 minutes | **Servings: 4** |
| --- | --- | --- |

Ingredients:

- ✓ 1 tablespoon extra virgin olive oil
- ✓ - 2 red peppers, seeded and finely chopped
- ✓ - 1 yellow onion, finely chopped
- ✓ - 2 cloves of garlic, finely chopped
- ✓ - 1 teaspoon ground cumin
- ✓ - ½ teaspoon ground turmeric

Ingredients:

- ✓ - ¼ teaspoon ground cinnamon
- ✓ - ¼ teaspoon ground ginger
- ✓ - 1 1/2 pounds ground lean lamb - Salt, to taste
- ✓ - 1 can diced tomatoes
- ✓ - 2 tablespoons harissa
- ✓ - 1 cup water - Fresh chopped cilantro, for garnish

Directions:

❖ In a large skillet, heat the oil over medium-high heat. Add the bell bell pepper, onion and garlic and sauté for about 5 minutes. Add the spices and sauté for about 1 minute. Add the lamb and salt and cook about 5 minutes, breaking it up into pieces.

❖ Add the tomatoes, harissa and water and bring to a boil. Reduce the heat to low and simmer, covered for about 1 hour. Serve hot while using the harissa garnish.

| 64) PAN-FRIED LAMB CHOPS | | |
|---|---|---|
| **Preparation Time**: 10 minutes | **Cooking Time**: 4-6 minutes | **Servings**: 4 |

Ingredients:

- ✓ 4 cloves of garlic, peeled - Salt, to taste
- ✓ - 1 teaspoon black mustard seeds, finely crushed
- ✓ - 2 teaspoons ground cumin
- ✓ - 1 teaspoon ground ginger

Ingredients:

- ✓ - 1 teaspoon ground coriander
- ✓ - ½ teaspoon ground cinnamon - Fresh ground black pepper, to taste.
- ✓ - 1 tablespoon coconut oil
- ✓ - 8 medium lamb chops, sliced

Directions:

- ❖ Place the garlic cloves on a cutting board and sprinkle with a little salt. Using a knife, crush the garlic until it forms a paste. In a bowl, mix together the garlic paste and spices.

- ❖ With a clear, crisp knife, make 3-4 cuts on both sides in the chops. Generously rub the chops with the garlic mixture. In a large skillet, melt the butter over medium heat. Add chops and cook for about 2-3 minutes per side or until desired doneness.

| 65) LAMB AND PINEAPPLE KEBAB | | |
|---|---|---|
| **Preparation Time**: 15 minutes | **Cooking Time**: 10 minutes | **Servings**: 4-6 |

Ingredients:

- ✓ 1 large pineapple, cut into 1½-inch cubes, split
- ✓ - 1 piece fresh ginger (½ inch), chopped
- ✓ - 2 cloves garlic, chopped - Salt, to taste

Ingredients:

- ✓
- ✓ - 16- to 24-ounce lamb shoulder steak, cut and diced into 1½-inch cubes –
- ✓ Fresh mint leaves from a bunch
- ✓ - Cinnamon powder, to taste

Directions:

- ❖ In a blender, add about 1 1/2 servings of pineapple, the ginger, garlic, and salt, and blend until smooth. Transfer the amalgam to a large bowl. Add chops and coat generously with mixture.

- ❖ Refrigerate to marinate for about 1-2 hours. Preheat grill to medium heat. Grease the grill grate. Thread lam, remaining pineapple, and mint leaves onto pre-soaked wooden skewers. Grill skewers for about 10 minutes, turning occasionally.

## 66) SPICED PORK ONE

| **Preparation Time**: 15 minutes | **Cooking Time**: 60 minutes | **Servings**: 6 |
|---|---|---|

Ingredients:

- ✓  1 (2-inch) piece of fresh ginger, chopped
- ✓  - 5-10 cloves of garlic, chopped
- ✓  - 1 teaspoon ground cumin
- ✓  - ½ teaspoon ground turmeric
- ✓  1 tablespoon ground hot paprika
- ✓  - 1 tablespoon red pepper flakes - Salt, to taste
- ✓  - 2 tablespoons cider vinegar
- ✓  - 2 pounds pork shoulder, chopped and diced
- ✓  1½ inches

Ingredients:

- ✓  - 2 cups domestic hot water, divided
- ✓  - 1 (1 inch wide) ball of tamarind pulp
- ✓  - ¼ cup olive oil
- ✓  - 1 teaspoon black mustard seeds, crushed
- ✓  - 4 green cardamoms
- ✓  - 5 whole cloves
- ✓  - 1 (3 inch) cinnamon stick
- ✓  - 1 cup onion, finely chopped
- ✓  - 1 large red bell pepper, seeded and chopped

Directions:

- ❖  In a food processor, add the ginger, garlic, cumin, turmeric, paprika, red pepper flakes, salt, and apple cider vinegar and pulse until smooth. Transfer the amalgam to a large bowl. Add the pork and coat generously with the mixture.
- ❖  Set aside, covered for about an hour at room temperature. In a bowl, add 1 cup hot water and tamarind and set aside until water cools. Using your hands, mash the tamarind to extract the pulp .

- ❖  Add the remaining cup of hot water and stir until well combined. Through a fine sieve, strain the tamarind juice into a bowl. In a large skillet, heat the oil over medium-high heat. Add the mustard seeds, green cardamoms, cloves and cinnamon stick and sauté for about 4 minutes.
- ❖  Add the onion and sauté for about 5 minutes. Add the pork and sauté for about 6 minutes. Add the tamarind juice and bring to a boil. Reduce heat to medium-low and simmer for 1 1/2 hours. Stir in bell bell pepper and cook for about 7 minutes.

## 67) PORK CHOPS IN CREAMY SAUCE

| **Preparation Time**: 15 minutes | **Cooking Time**: 14 minutes | **Servings**: 4 |
|---|---|---|

Ingredients:

- ✓  2 garlic cloves, chopped
- ✓  - 1 small jalapeño bell pepper, chopped
- ✓  - ¼ cup fresh cilantro leaves
- ✓  - 1½ teaspoons turmeric powder, divided
- ✓  - 1 tablespoon fish sauce
- ✓  - 2 tablespoons fresh lime juice

Ingredients:

- ✓  - 1 can coconut milk (13½-ounce)
- ✓  - 4 pork chops (½-inch thick)
- ✓  - Salt, to taste
- ✓  - 1 tablespoon coconut oil
- ✓  - 1 shallot, finely chopped

Directions:

- ❖  In a blender, add the garlic, jalapeño bell pepper, cilantro, 1 teaspoon ground turmeric, fish sauce, lime juice, and coconut milk, and blend until smooth.
- ❖  Sprinkle the pork evenly with the salt and remaining turmeric. In a skillet, melt the butter over medium-high heat. Add the shallots and sauté about 1 minute. Add the chops and cook for about 2 minutes per side. Transfer chops to a bowl. Add the coconut mixture and bring to a boil.

- ❖  Reduce heat to medium and simmer, stirring occasionally for about 5 minutes. Stir in the pork chops and cook for about 3-4 minutes. Serve hot.

## 68) DECENT BEEF AND ONION STEW

| **Preparation Time**: 10 minutes | **Cooking Time**: 1-2 hours | **Servings**: 4 |
| --- | --- | --- |

Ingredients:

- ✓ 2 pounds lean beef, cubed
- ✓ 3 pounds shallots, peeled
- ✓ 5 garlic cloves, peeled, whole
- ✓ 3 tablespoons tomato paste

Ingredients:

- ✓ 1 bay leaf
- ✓ ¼ cup olive oil
- ✓ 3 tablespoons lemon juice

Directions:

❖ Take a stew pot and place it over medium heat. Add the olive oil and let it heat up. Add the meat and let it brown.

❖ Add the remaining ingredients and cover with water. Bring everything to a boil. Reduce the heat to low and cover the pot. Simmer for 1-2 hours until meat is cooked through. Serve hot!

## 69) BEEF SAUTEED WITH ZUCCHINI AND CILANTRO

| **Preparation Time**: 10 minutes | **Cooking Time**: 10 minutes | **Servings**: 4 |
| --- | --- | --- |

Ingredients:

- ✓ 10 ounces beef, cut into 1-2-inch strips
- ✓ 1 zucchini, cut into 2-inch strips
- ✓ ¼ cup parsley, chopped

Ingredients:

- ✓ 3 cloves garlic, chopped
- ✓ 2 tablespoons tamari sauce
- ✓ 4 tablespoons avocado oil

Directions:

❖ Add 2 tablespoons avocado oil to a skillet over high heat. Place the beef strips in and sauté for a few minutes over high heat.

❖ Once the meat is brown, add the zucchini strips and sauté until tender. Once tender, add the tamari sauce, garlic, parsley and let them sit for a few more minutes. Serve immediately and enjoy!

## 70) WALNUT AND ASPARAGUS DELIGHT

| **Preparation Time**: 5 minutes | **Cooking Time**: 5 minutes | **Servings**: 4 |
| --- | --- | --- |

Ingredients:

- ✓ 1 ½ tablespoons olive oil
- ✓ ¾ pound asparagus, chopped

Ingredients:

- ✓ ¼ cup walnuts, chopped Sunflower seeds and pepper to taste

Directions:

❖ Place a skillet over medium heat, add the olive oil and let it heat up. Add asparagus and saute for 5 minutes until browned.

❖ Season with sunflower seeds and pepper. Remove from heat. Add walnuts and toss to combine. Serve hot!

## 71) BEEF SOUP

| **Preparation Time**: 10 minutes | **Cooking Time:** 40 minutes | **Servings: 4** |
|---|---|---|

Ingredients:

- ✓ 1 pound ground beef, lean
- ✓ 1 cup mixed vegetables, frozen
- ✓ 1 yellow onion, chopped

Ingredients:

- ✓ 6 cups vegetable broth
- ✓ 1 cup low-fat cream
- ✓ Pepper to taste

Directions:

- ❖ Take a pot and add all ingredients except heavy cream, salt and black pepper. Bring to a boil. Reduce heat to a simmer.

- ❖ Cook for 40 minutes. Once cooked, heat the heavy cream. Then add once the soup is cooked. Blend the soup until smooth using an immersion blender. Season with salt and black pepper. Serve and enjoy!

## 72) CLEANED CHICKEN AND MUSHROOM STEW

| **Preparation Time**: 10 minutes | **Cooking Time:** 35 minutes | **Servings: 4** |
|---|---|---|

Ingredients:

- ✓ 4 chicken breast halves, cut into bite-sized pieces
- ✓ 1 pound mushrooms, sliced (5-6 cups)
- ✓ 1 bunch onion, chopped

Ingredients:

- ✓ 4 tablespoons olive oil
- ✓ 1 teaspoon thyme Sunflower seeds and pepper as needed

Directions:

- ❖ Take a large deep skillet and place it over medium-high heat. Add the oil and let it heat up. Add the chicken and cook for 4-5 minutes per side until lightly browned.

- ❖ Add the spring onions and mushrooms, season with the sunflower seeds and pepper to your taste. Stir. Cover with the lid and bring the mixture to a boil. Reduce heat and simmer for 25 minutes. Serve.

## 73) ZUCCHINI ZOODLES WITH CHICKEN AND BASIL

| **Preparation Time**: 10 minutes | **Cooking Time:** 10 minutes | **Servings: 2** |
|---|---|---|

Ingredients:

- ✓ 2 chicken fillets, diced
- ✓ 2 tablespoons ghee
- ✓ 1 pound tomatoes, diced
- ✓ ½ cup basil, chopped

Ingredients:

- ✓ ¼ cup coconut milk
- ✓ 1 garlic clove, peeled, chopped
- ✓ 1 zucchini, chopped

Directions:

- ❖ Fry the diced chicken in the ghee until no longer pink. Add the tomatoes and season with the sunflower seeds. Simmer and reduce the liquid. Prepare your Zucchini Zoodles by chopping the zucchini in a food processor.

- ❖ Add the basil, garlic, coconut milk and almonds to the chicken and cook for a few minutes. Add half of the Zucchini Zoodles to a bowl and top with the creamy tomato basil chicken. Enjoy!

## 74) THE GOODNESS OF BREADED CHICKEN WITH ALMONDS

| **Preparation Time**: 15 minutes | **Cooking Time:** 15 minutes | **Servings: 3** |
| --- | --- | --- |

Ingredients:

- ✓ 2 large chicken breasts, boneless and skinless
- ✓ 1/3 cup lemon juice
- ✓ 1 ½ cups seasoned almond flour

Ingredients:

- ✓ 2 tablespoons coconut oil Lemon pepper, to taste
- ✓ Parsley for garnish

Directions:

- ❖ Cut the chicken breast in half. Pound each half until ¼ inch thick. Take a skillet and place it over medium heat, add the oil and heat it up. Dip each slice of chicken breast into the lemon juice and let it sit for 2 minutes.

- ❖ Flip and let the other side rest for 2 minutes. Transfer to almond flour and coat both sides. Add the coated chicken to the oil and fry for 4 minutes per side, making sure to liberally sprinkle the lemon pepper.
- ❖ Transfer to a paper-lined sheet and repeat until all chicken is fried. Garnish with parsley and enjoy!

## 75) PORK CHOPS WITH ALMOND BUTTER

| **Preparation Time**: 5 minutes | **Cooking Time:** 25 minutes | **Servings: 2** |
| --- | --- | --- |

Ingredients:

- ✓ 1 tablespoon almond butter, divided
- ✓ 2 boneless pork chops Pepper to taste

Ingredients:

- ✓ 1 tablespoon dry, low-fat, low-sodium Italian seasoning
- ✓ 1 tablespoon olive oil

Directions:

- ❖ preheat oven to 350 degrees F. Pat pork chops dry with a paper towel and place in a baking dish. Season with pepper and Italian seasoning.

- ❖ Drizzle pork chops with olive oil. Top each chop with ½ tablespoon almond butter. Bake for 25 minutes. Transfer pork chops to two plates and top with almond butter. Serve and enjoy!

## 76) HEALTHY MEDITERRANEAN LAMB CHOPS

| **Preparation Time**: 10 minutes | **Cooking Time:** 10 minutes | **Servings: 4** |
| --- | --- | --- |

Ingredients:

- ✓ 4 lamb shoulder chops,
- ✓ 8 ounces each
- ✓ 2 tablespoons Dijon mustard

Ingredients:

- ✓ 2 tablespoons balsamic vinegar
- ✓ ½ cup olive oil
- ✓ 2 tablespoons chopped fresh basil

Directions:

- ❖ Dry the lamb chops with a kitchen towel and place them on a shallow glass baking dish. Take a bowl and whisk in Dijon mustard, balsamic vinegar, and pepper and mix well.
- ❖ Very slowly whisk the oil into the marinade until the mixture is smooth Stir in the basil. Pour the marinade over the lamb chops and stir to coat both sides well. Cover the ribs and let them marinate for 1-4 hours (in a cool place).

- ❖ Remove the ribs and let them sit for 30 minutes to allow the temperature to reach a normal level. Preheat grill to medium heat and add oil to grill.
- ❖ Grill the lamb chops for 5-10 minutes per side until both sides are golden brown. When the center reads 145 degrees F, the ribs are ready, serve and enjoy!

## 77) DUCK BREAST WITH BROWN BUTTER

| **Preparation Time**: 5 minutes | **Cooking Time**: 25 minutes | **Servings: 3** |
|---|---|---|

Ingredients:

✓ 1 whole
✓ 6-ounce duck breast, with skin Pepper to taste
✓ 1 head of radicchio, 4 ounces, coreless

Ingredients:

✓ ¼ cup unsalted butter
✓ 6 fresh sage leaves, sliced

Directions:

❖ Preheat oven to 400 degrees F. Dry duck breast with paper towel. Season with the pepper. Place the duck breast in a skillet and place over medium heat, sear for 3-4 minutes each side. Turn the breast and transfer the pan to the oven. Roast for 10 minutes (uncovered).

❖ Cut the radicchio in half. Remove and discard the woody white core and thinly slice the leaves. Keep them aside. Remove the pan from the oven. Transfer the duck breast, fat side up, to the cutting board and let it rest.

❖ Reheat the skillet over medium heat. Add the unsalted butter and sage and cook for 3-4 minutes. Cut the duck into 6 equal slices. Divide the radicchio between 2 plates, top with the duck breast slices and drizzle with browned butter and sage. Enjoy!

## 78) CAULIFLOWER BREAD STICK

| **Preparation Time**: 10 minutes | **Cooking Time**: 48 minutes | **Servings: 5** |
|---|---|---|

Ingredients:

✓ 1 cup cashew/ricotta kite cheese
✓ 1 tablespoon organic almond butter
✓ 1 whole egg
✓ ½ teaspoon Italian seasoning
✓ ¼ teaspoon red pepper flakes

Ingredients:

✓ 1/8 teaspoon kosher sunflower seeds
✓ 2 cups cauliflower rice, cooked for 3 minutes in the microwave
✓ 3 teaspoons garlic, minced
✓ Parmesan, grated

Directions:

❖ Preheat oven to 350 degrees F. Add almond butter to a small skillet and melt over low heat Add red pepper flakes, garlic to almond butter and cook for 2-3 minutes. Add the garlic and almond butter mixture to the bowl with the cooked cauliflower and add the Italian seasoning. Season with the sunflower seeds and toss, refrigerate for 10 minutes.

❖ Add the cheese and eggs to the bowl and mix. Place a layer of parchment paper in the bottom of a 9 x 9 baking dish and grease with cooking spray, add the egg and mozzarella mixture to the cauliflower mixture.

❖ Add the mixture to the baking dish and smooth it out to a thin layer with the palms of your hand. Bake for 30 minutes, remove from oven and top with a few shakes of parmesan and mozzarella cheese. Bake for an additional 8 minutes. Enjoy!

## 79) CHICKEN WITH CHIPOTLE LETTUCE

| **Preparation Time**: 10 minutes | **Cooking Time**: 25 minutes | **Servings: 6** |
|---|---|---|

Ingredients:

✓ 1 pound chicken breast, cut into strips
✓ Drizzle with olive oil
✓ 1 red onion, finely sliced
✓ 14 ounces tomatoes
✓ 1 teaspoon chipotle, chopped

Ingredients:

✓ ½ teaspoon cumin
✓ Lettuce as needed
✓ Fresh cilantro leaves
✓ Jalapeno chiles, sliced
✓ Fresh tomato slices for garnish Lime wedge

❖ Take a non-stick skillet and place it over medium heat. Add the oil and heat it up. Add the chicken and cook until it turns brown. Keep the chicken aside. Add the tomatoes, sugar, chipotle, and cumin to the same pan and simmer for 25 minutes until you have a nice sauce.

❖ Add the chicken to the sauce and cook for 5 minutes. Transfer the mixture to another place. Use lettuce strips to take a portion of the mixture and serve with a squeeze of lemon. Enjoy!

## 80) CREAMED CORN DISH

| **Preparation Time**: 10 minutes | **Cooking Time**: 4 hour | **Servings: 3** |
|---|---|---|

| Ingredients: | Ingredients: |
|---|---|
| ✓ 3 cups corn<br>✓ 2 ounces cream cheese, cubed<br>✓ 2 tablespoons milk<br>✓ 2 tablespoons whipping cream | ✓ 2 tablespoons melted butter<br>✓ Salt and pepper to taste<br>✓ 1 tablespoon green onion, chopped |
| Directions:<br><br>❖ Add the corn, cream cheese, milk, whipping cream, butter, salt and pepper to your Slow Cooker. Give it a good stir to mix everything well. | ❖ Put the lid on and cook on LOW for 4 hours. Divide the mixture between serving plates. Serve and enjoy! |

## 81) ETHIOPIAN CABBAGE DELIGHT

| **Preparation Time**: 15 minutes | **Cooking Time**: 6-8 hour | **Servings: 6** |
|---|---|---|

| Ingredients: | Ingredients: |
|---|---|
| ✓ ½ cup water<br>✓ 1 head of kale, chopped and shredded<br>✓ 1 pound sweet potatoes, peeled and shredded<br>✓ 3 carrots, peeled and shredded<br>✓ 1 onion, sliced | ✓ 1 teaspoon extra virgin olive oil<br>✓ ½ teaspoon turmeric powder<br>✓ ½ teaspoon cumin powder<br>✓ ¼ teaspoon ginger powder |
| Directions:<br><br>❖ Add water to your Slow Cooker. Take a medium bowl and add cabbage, carrots, sweet potatoes, onion and mix. | ❖ Add the olive oil, turmeric, ginger, cumin and stir until the vegetables are completely coated. Transfer the vegetable mix to your Slow Cooker.<br>❖ Cover and cook on LOW for 6-8 hours. Serve and enjoy! |

## 82) FRESH HARMONY OF APPLES AND CARROTS

| **Preparation Time**: 10 minutes | **Cooking Time**: 10 minutes | **Servings: 6** |
|---|---|---|

| Ingredients: | Ingredients: |
|---|---|
| ✓ 1 cup apple juice<br>✓ 1 pound baby carrots | ✓ 1 tablespoon cornstarch<br>✓ 1 tablespoon chopped mint |
| Directions:<br><br>❖ Add the apple juice, carrots, cornstarch and mint to your Instant Pot. Stir and close the lid. | ❖ Cook on high pressure for 10 minutes. Perform a quick release. Divide the mix among plates and serve. Enjoy! |

| *83)* **BLACK PEAS AND SPINACH DISH** | | |
| --- | --- | --- |
| **Preparation Time**: 10 minutes | **Cooking Time:** 8 hours | **Servings: 4** |

Ingredients:

- ✓ 1 cup black peas, soaked overnight and drained
- ✓ 2 cups low-sodium vegetable broth
- ✓ 1 can (15 ounces) tomatoes, diced with juice
- ✓ 8 ounces ham, chopped
- ✓ 1 onion, chopped
- ✓ 2 cloves garlic, chopped

Ingredients:

- ✓ 1 teaspoon dried oregano
- ✓ 1 teaspoon salt
- ✓ ½ teaspoon freshly ground black pepper
- ✓ ½ teaspoon ground mustard
- ✓ 1 bay leaf

Directions:

- ❖ Add the ingredients listed in your Slow Cooker and stir. Put the lid on and cook on LOW for 8 hours. Discard the bay leaf. Serve and enjoy!

| *84)* **CABBAGE AND APPLES IN SWEET AND SOUR SAUCE** | | |
| --- | --- | --- |
| **Preparation Time**: 15 minutes | **Cooking Time:** 8 hours | **Servings: 4** |

Ingredients:

- ✓ ¼ cup honey
- ✓ ¼ cup apple cider vinegar
- ✓ 2 tablespoons orange-garlic sauce
- ✓ 1 teaspoon sea salt

Ingredients:

- ✓ 3 tart sweet apples, peeled, pitted and sliced
- ✓ 2 heads of collard greens, pitted and chopped
- ✓ 1 sweet red onion, thinly sliced

Directions:

- ❖ Take a small bowl and whisk together the honey, orange garlic and chili sauce, and vinegar. Mix well. Add the honey mixture, apples, onion and cabbage to your Slow Cooker and stir.

- ❖ Close the lid and cook on LOW for 8 hours. Serve and enjoy!

| *85)* **GARLIC SAUCE WITH ORANGE AND CHILI PEPPER** | | |
| --- | --- | --- |
| **Preparation Time**: 15 minutes | **Cooking Time:** 8 hours | **Servings: 5** |

Ingredients:

- ✓ ½ cup apple cider vinegar
- ✓ 4 pounds red jalapeno peppers, stems, seeds and ribs removed, chopped
- ✓ 10 cloves garlic, chopped
- ✓ ½ cup tomato paste

Ingredients:

- ✓ Juice of 1 orange peel
- ✓ ½ cup honey
- ✓ 2 tablespoons soy sauce
- ✓ 2 teaspoons salt

- ❖ Add the vinegar, garlic, peppers, tomato paste, orange juice, honey, zest, soy sauce and salt to your Slow Cooker. Stir and close the lid. Cook on LOW for 8 hours. Use as needed

## 86) VEGETABLE BROTH FOR EVERY DAY

| **Preparation Time**: 5 minutes | **Cooking Time**: 8-12 hours | **Servings: 10** |
| --- | --- | --- |

Ingredients:

- ✓ 2 celery stalks (with leaves), quartered
- ✓ 4 ounces mushrooms, with stalks
- ✓ 2 carrots, unpeeled and quartered
- ✓ 1 onion, unpeeled, quartered pole to pole
- ✓ 1 garlic head, unpeeled, halved in center

Ingredients:

- ✓ 2 sprigs fresh thyme
- ✓ 10 peppercorns
- ✓ ½ teaspoon salt
- ✓ Enough water to fill 3 quarts of Slow Cooker

Directions:

- ❖ Add celery, mushrooms, onion, carrots, garlic, thyme, salt, pepper and water to pot over low heat. Stir and cover.

- ❖ Cook on LOW for 8-12 hours. Strain broth through a fine mesh cloth/wire mesh and discard solids. Use as needed.

## 87) CARAMELIZED PORK CHOPS AND ONION

| **Preparation Time**: 5 minutes | **Cooking Time**: 40 minutes | **Servings: 4** |
| --- | --- | --- |

Ingredients:

- ✓ Roast 4-pound beef
- ✓ 4 ounces green chile, minced
- ✓ 2 tablespoons chili powder

Ingredients:

- ✓ ½ teaspoon dried oregano
- ✓ ½ teaspoon cumin, ground
- ✓ 2 cloves garlic, minced

Directions:

- ❖ Rub the chops with a seasoning of 1 teaspoon pepper and 2 teaspoons sunflower seeds. Take a skillet and place it over medium heat, add the oil and let the oil heat up Brown the seasoned chops on both sides.

- ❖ Add the water and onion to the skillet and cover, lower the heat to low and simmer for 20 minutes. Turn the chops over and season with more sunflower seeds and pepper. Cover and cook until the water evaporates completely and the beer shows a slightly brown consistency.
- ❖ Remove chops and serve with a caramelized onion garnish. Serve and enjoy!

## 88) APPLE PIE CRACKERS

| **Preparation Time**: 10 minutes | **Cooking Time**: 2 hours | **Servings: 100 crackers** |
| --- | --- | --- |

Ingredients:

- ✓ 2 tablespoons + 2 teaspoons avocado oil
- ✓ 1 medium Granny Smith apple, coarsely chopped
- ✓ ¼ cup erythritol
- ✓ 1/4 cup sunflower seeds, coarsely ground
- ✓ 1 ¾ cup flax seeds, coarsely ground

Ingredients:

- ✓ 1/8 teaspoon clove powder
- ✓ 1/8 teaspoon cardamom powder
- ✓ 3 tablespoons nutmeg
- ✓ ¼ teaspoon ginger powder

Directions:

- ❖ Preheat oven to 225 degrees F. Line two baking sheets with baking paper and set aside. Add the oil, apple, and erythritol to a bowl and mix.

- ❖ Transfer to a food processor and add remaining ingredients, process until combined. Transfer batter to baking sheets, spread evenly and cut into crackers. Bake for 1 hour, turn and bake for another hour. Let them cool and serve. Enjoy!

## 89) GROUND BEEF AND VEGETABLE CURRY

| **Preparation Time**: 15 minutes | **Cooking Time**: 36 minutes | **Servings**: 6-8 |
|---|---|---|

Ingredients:

- ✓ 2-3 tablespoons coconut oil
- ✓ - 1 cup onion, chopped
- ✓ - 1 clove garlic, chopped
- ✓ - 1 pound lean ground beef –
- ✓ 1½ tablespoons curry powder
- ✓ - 1/8 teaspoon ginger powder

Ingredients:

- ✓ - 1/8 teaspoon cinnamon powder
- ✓ - 1/8 teaspoon turmeric powder
- ✓ - Salt, to taste
- ✓ - 2½-3 cups tomatoes, finely chopped
- ✓ - 2½-3 cups fresh peas, shelled
- ✓ - 2 sweet potatoes, peeled and chopped

Directions:

- ❖ In a large skillet, melt the coconut oil over medium heat. Add the onion and garlic and sauté for about 4-5 minutes. Add the beef and cook for about 4-5 minutes.

- ❖ Add the curry powder and spices and cook for about 1 minute. Add the tomatoes, peas and sweet potato and bring to a boil over low heat. Simmer, covered for about 25 minutes.

## 90) HONEY GLAZED BEEF

| **Preparation Time**: quarter hour | **Cooking Time**: 12 minutes | **Servings**: 2-3 |
|---|---|---|

Ingredients:

- ✓ 2 Tablespoons arrowroot flour - Salt and freshly ground black pepper, to taste
- ✓ - 1 lb. beefsteak, cut into ¼ inch thick slices
- ✓ - ½ cup plus 1 tbsp. coconut oil, divided –
- ✓ 2 cloves minced garlic
- ✓ - 1 teaspoon ground ginger

Ingredients:

- ✓ - Pinch of red pepper flakes, crushed
- ✓ - 1/3 cup organic honey
- ✓ - ½ cup beef broth
- ✓ - ½ cup coconut aminos
- ✓ - 3 shallots, chopped

Directions:

- ❖ In a bowl, mix together the arrowroot flour, salt and black pepper. Coat the beef slices in the arrowroot flour mixture evenly after which get rid of the excess mixture. Set aside for about 10-15 minutes. For the sauce in a skillet, melt 1 tablespoon of coconut oil over medium heat.
- ❖ Add the garlic, ginger powder and red pepper flakes and sauté for about 1 minute. Add the honey, broth and coconut amino acid and stir to mix well. Increase the heat to high and cook, stirring constantly for about 3 minutes. Remove from heat and set aside. In a large skillet, melt the remaining coconut oil over medium heat. Add beef and stir-fry about 2-3 minutes.

- ❖ Transfer beef to a paper towel-lined plate to drain. Remove the oil from the pan and return the beef to the pan. Sauté for about 1 minute. Add the honey sauce and cook for about 3 minutes. Add the shallot and cook for about 1 minute. Serve hot.

## 91) ROAST LAMB WITH SPINACH

| **Preparation Time**: quarter hour | **Cooking Time:** 55 minutes | **Servings: 6** |
| --- | --- | --- |

Ingredients:

- ✓ 2 tablespoons coconut oil
- ✓ - 2 pounds lamb necks, trimmed and cut into 2-inch pieces crosswise
- ✓ - Salt, to taste
- ✓ - 2 medium onions, chopped
- ✓ - 3 tablespoons fresh ginger, chopped
- ✓ - 4 cloves garlic, chopped
- ✓ - 2 tablespoons ground coriander
- ✓ - 1 tablespoon ground cumin
- ✓ - 1 teaspoon ground turmeric

Ingredients:

- ✓ - ¼ cup coconut milk
- ✓ - ½ cup tomatoes, chopped
- ✓ - 2 cups boiling water
- ✓ - 30 ounces frozen spinach, thawed and squeezed
- ✓ - 1½ tablespoons garam masala
- ✓ - 1 tablespoon fresh lemon juice
- ✓ - Freshly ground black pepper, to taste

Directions:

❖ Preheat oven to 300 degrees F. In a substantial Dutch oven, melt the coconut oil over medium-high heat. Add the lamb necks and sprinkle with salt. Sauté about 4-5 minutes or until completely browned.

❖ Transfer the lamb to a plate and lower the heat to medium. In the same pan, add the onion and sauté for about 10 minutes. Add the ginger, garlic and spices and sauté for about 1 minute.

❖ Add the coconut milk and tomatoes and cook about 3-4 minutes. Using an immersion blender, blend the mixture until smooth. Add the lamb, boiling water and salt and bring to a boil. Cover the pot and transfer to the oven.

❖ Bake about 2 1/2 hours. Now, remove the pan from the oven and place on medium heat. Stir in the spinach and garam masala and cook for about 3-5 minutes. Add the fresh lemon juice, salt and black pepper and remove from heat. Serve hot.

## 92) GRILLED SHOULDER OF LAMB

| **Preparation Time**: 10 minutes | **Cooking Time:** 8-10 minutes | **Servings: 10** |
| --- | --- | --- |

Ingredients:

- ✓ 2 tablespoons fresh ginger, chopped
- ✓ - 2 tablespoons garlic, chopped
- ✓ - ¼ cup fresh lemongrass, chopped
- ✓ - ¼ cup fresh orange juice

Ingredients:

- ✓ - ¼ cup coconut aminos
- ✓ - freshly ground black pepper, to taste
- ✓ - 2 pounds lamb shoulder, chopped

Directions:

❖ In a bowl, mix all ingredients except lamb shoulder. In a baking dish, mash the lamb shoulder and generously coat the lamb with half of the marinade mixture. Reserve the remaining mixture. Refrigerate to marinate overnight.

❖ Preheat the broiler in the oven. Place a rack inside a broiler pan and arrange about 4-5 inches from the heating unit. Remove lamb shoulder from refrigerator and remove excess marinade. Bake for about 4-5 minutes on both sides. Serve with all the reserved marinade as a sauce.

## 93) LAMB BURGERS WITH AVOCADO SAUCE

| **Preparation Time**: 20 minutes | **Cooking Time:** 10 minutes | **Servings: 4-6** |
|---|---|---|

**Ingredients:**

For the burgers:
- ✓ - 1 (2 inch) piece of fresh ginger, grated
- ✓ - 1 pound of lean ground lamb
- ✓ - 1 medium onion, grated
- ✓ - 2 cloves of garlic, minced
- ✓ - 1 bunch of fresh mint leaves, finely chopped
- ✓ - 2 teaspoons ground coriander
- ✓ - 2 teaspoons ground cumin
- ✓ - ½ teaspoon ground allspice
- ✓ - ½ teaspoon ground cinnamon
- ✓ - Salt and freshly ground black pepper, to taste
- ✓ - 1 tablespoon essential olive oil

**Ingredients:**

For the sauce:
- ✓ - 3 small cucumbers, peeled and grated
- ✓ - 1 avocado, peeled, pitted and chopped
- ✓ - ½ of garlic oil, crushed
- ✓ - 2 tablespoons fresh lemon juice
- ✓ - 2 tablespoons olive oil
- ✓ - 2 tablespoons fresh dill, finely chopped
- ✓ - 2 tablespoons chives, finely chopped
- ✓ - Salt and freshly ground black pepper, to taste

**Directions:**

❖ Preheat oven rack. Lightly grease a broiler pan. For burgers in a large bowl, squeeze ginger juice. Add the remaining ingredients and mix until well combined. Make equal-sized burgers from your mixture.

❖ Place the burgers in a broiler pan and cook about 5 minutes per side. Meanwhile for the dip squeeze the juice from the cucumbers into a bowl. In a blender, add the avocado, garlic, lemon juice and oil and blend until smooth.

❖ Transfer the avocado mixture to a bowl. Add the remaining ingredients and stir to mix. Serve the burgers with the avocado sauce.

## 94) PORK WITH PINEAPPLE

| **Preparation Time**: 15 minutes | **Cooking Time:** 14 minutes | **Servings: 4** |
|---|---|---|

**Ingredients:**

- ✓ 2 tablespoons coconut oil
- ✓ - 1½ pound pork
- ✓ 10 derloin, trimmed and cut into bite-size pieces
- ✓ - 1 onion, chopped
- ✓ - 2 cloves garlic, chopped
- ✓ - 1 (1-inch) piece fresh ginger, chopped

**Ingredients:**

- ✓ - 20-ounce pineapple, chopped
- ✓ - 1 large red bell bell pepper, seeded and chopped
- ✓ - ¼ cup fresh pineapple juice
- ✓ - ¼ cup coconut aminos
- ✓ - Salt and freshly ground black pepper, to taste

**Directions:**

❖ In a substantial skillet, melt the coconut oil over high heat. Add pork and sauté about 4-5 minutes. Transfer pork to a bowl. In the exact same pan, heat the remaining oil over medium heat.

❖ Add the onion, garlic and ginger and sauté for about 2 minutes. Add the pineapple and bell bell pepper and sauté for about 3 minutes.

❖ Add the pork, pineapple juice and coconut amino acid and cook for about 3-4 minutes. Serve hot.

## 95) PORK CHOPS GLAZED WITH PEACH

| **Preparation Time**: quarter hour | **Cooking Time**: 16 minutes | **Servings: 2** |
|---|---|---|

Ingredients:

- ✓ 2 boneless pork chops
- ✓ - Salt and freshly ground black pepper, to taste
- ✓ - 1 ripe yellow peach, peeled, pitted, chopped and split
- ✓ - 1 tablespoon organic olive oil
- ✓ - 2 tablespoons shallots, chopped
- ✓ - 2 tablespoons garlic, minced

Ingredients:

- ✓ - 2 tablespoons fresh ginger, minced
- ✓ - 1 tablespoon organic honey –
- ✓ 1 tablespoon balsamic vinegar
- ✓ - 1 tablespoon coconut aminos
- ✓ - ¼ tablespoon red pepper flakes, crushed
- ✓ - ¼ cup water

Directions:

- ❖ Sprinkle pork chops generously with salt and black pepper. In a blender, add 1/2 of the peach and pulse until it forms a puree. Reserve the remaining peach. In a skillet, heat oil over medium heat.
- ❖ Add the shallots and sauté about 1-2 minutes. Add the garlic and ginger and sauté about 1 minute. Add the remaining ingredients and lower the heat to medium-low. Bring to a boil and simmer about 4-5 minutes or until a sticky glaze forms. Remove from heat and reserve 1/3 with the glaze and keep aside. Coat the chops with the remaining glaze. Heat a nonstick skillet over medium-high heat.

❖ Add the chops and sear for about 4 minutes on both sides. Transfer chops to a plate and coat with all remaining glaze evenly. Top with reserved chopped peaches and serve.

## 96) BEEF WITH CARROTS AND BROCCOLI

| **Preparation Time**: 15 minutes | **Cooking Time**: 14 minutes | **Servings: 4** |
|---|---|---|

Ingredients:

- ✓ 2 tablespoons coconut oil, divided
- ✓ - 2 medium garlic cloves, minced
- ✓ - 1 pound sirloin steak, trimmed and cut into thin strips
- ✓ - Salt, to taste
- ✓ - ¼ cup chicken broth
- ✓ - 2 teaspoons fresh ginger, grated

Ingredients:

- ✓ - 1 tablespoon ground flaxseed
- ✓ - ½ teaspoon red pepper flakes, crushed
- ✓ - ¼ teaspoon freshly ground black pepper –
- ✓ 1 large carrot, peeled and thinly sliced
- ✓ - 2 cups broccoli florets
- ✓ - 1 medium shallot, thinly sliced

Directions:

- ❖ In a substantial skillet, heat 1 tablespoon oil over medium-high heat. Add garlic and sauté about 1 minute. Add the beef and salt and cook for about 4-5 minutes or until golden brown.

- ❖ Using a slotted spoon, transfer the beef to a bowl. Remove the liquid from the pan. In a bowl, mix together broth, ginger, flaxseed, red pepper flakes and black pepper. In a similar skillet, heat the remaining oil over medium heat.
- ❖ Add carrot, broccoli and ginger mixture and cook for about 3-4 minutes or until desired doneness. Add beef and shallots and cook for about 3-4 minutes.

# Chapter 4. DESSERTS

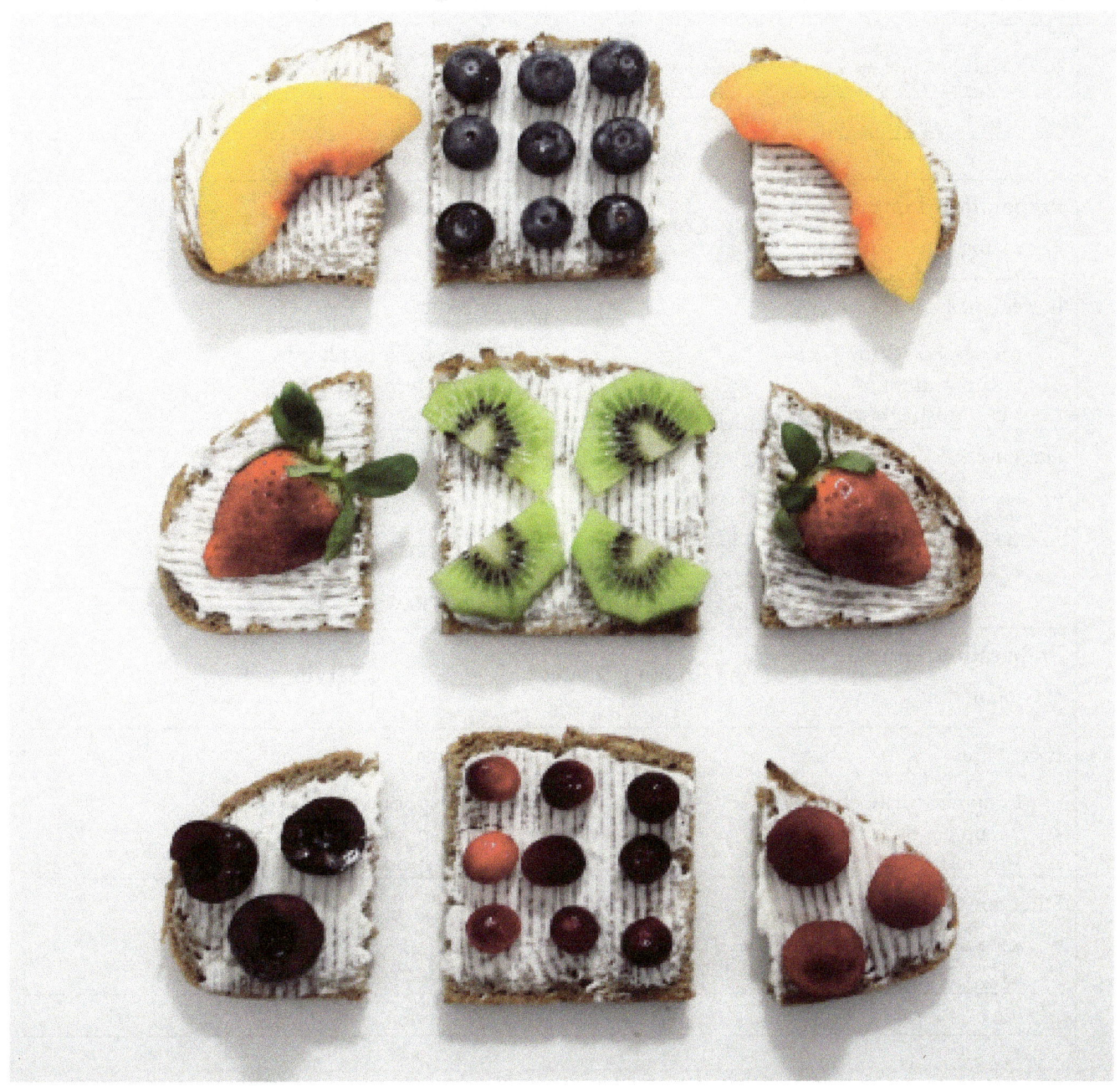

## 97) STRAWBERRY AND AVOCADO MEDLEY

| Preparation Time: | Cooking time: 5 minutes | Servings: 4 |
|---|---|---|

| Ingredients: | Ingredients: |
|---|---|
| ✓ 2 cups strawberries, cut in half<br>✓ 1 avocado, pitted and sliced | ✓ 2 tablespoons slivered almonds |

**Directions:**

❖ Place all ingredients in a mixing bowl. Stir to combine. Allow to cool in the refrigerator before serving.

## 98) HONEY AND BERRIES GRANITA

| Preparation Time: 10 minutes<br>+ freezing time | Cooking Time: | Servings: 4 |
|---|---|---|

| Ingredients: | Ingredients: |
|---|---|
| ✓ 1 teaspoon lemon juice<br>✓ ¼ cup honey<br>✓ 1 cup fresh strawberries | ✓ 1 cup fresh raspberries<br>✓ 1 cup fresh blueberries |

**Directions:**

❖ Bring 1 cup of water to a boil in a saucepan over high heat. Stir in honey until dissolved. Remove from heat and stir in berries and lemon juice; allow to cool.

❖ Once cooled, add mixture to a food processor and pulse until smooth. Transfer to a shallow glass and freeze for 1 hour. Stir with a fork and freeze for another 30 minutes. Repeat a couple of times. Serve in dessert dishes.

## 99) CHOCOLATE COVERED STRAWBERRIES

| Preparation Time: 15 minutes<br>+ cooling time | Cooking Time: | Servings: 4 |
|---|---|---|

| Ingredients: | Ingredients: |
|---|---|
| ✓ 1 cup chocolate chips<br>✓ ¼ cup coconut flakes<br>✓ 1 pound strawberries | ✓ ½ teaspoon vanilla extract<br>✓ ½ teaspoon nutmeg powder<br>✓ ¼ teaspoon salt |

**Directions:**

❖ Melt chocolate chips for 30 seconds. Remove and stir in vanilla, nutmeg and salt. Allow to cool for 2-3 minutes. Dip strawberries into chocolate and then into coconut chips.

❖ Place on a cookie sheet lined with wax paper and let sit for 30 minutes until the chocolate dries. Serve.

| *100)* | SUMMER FRUIT SORBET | |
|---|---|---|
| **Preparation Time**: 10 minutes + freezing time | **Cooking Time:** | **Servings: 4** |

Ingredients:

- ✓ ¼ cup honey
- ✓ 4 cups watermelon cubes

Ingredients:

- ✓ ¼ cup lemon juice
- ✓ 12 mint leaves to serve

Directions:

❖ In a food processor, blend the watermelon, honey and lemon juice to form a chunky puree. Transfer to a freezer-proof container and place in the freezer for 1 hour.

❖ Remove container and scrape with a fork. Place back in the freezer and repeat the process every half hour until the sorbet is completely frozen, about 4 hours. Distribute into bowls, garnish with mint leaves and serve.

| *101)* | HONEY PUDDING WITH KIWI | |
|---|---|---|
| **Preparation Time:** | **Cooking Time:** | **Servings:** |

Ingredients:

- ✓ 2 kiwis, halved and sliced
- ✓ 1 egg
- ✓ 2 ¼ cups milk

Ingredients:

- ✓ 2 kiwis, halved and sliced
- ✓ 1 egg
- ✓ 2 ¼ cups milk

Directions:

❖ In a bowl, beat egg with honey. Stir in 2 cups of milk and vanilla. Pour into a saucepan over medium heat and bring to a boil. Combine cornstarch and remaining milk in a bowl.

❖ Pour slowly into the pot and boil for 1 minute until thickened, stirring often. Divide among 4 cups and transfer to refrigerator. Add the kiwis and serve.

| *102)* | PEACH CAKE WITH WALNUTS AND RAISINS | |
|---|---|---|
| **Preparation Time**: 50 minutes + cooling time | **Cooking Time:** | **Servings: 6** |

Ingredients:

- ✓ 2 peaches, peeled and chopped
- ✓ ½ cup raisins, soaked
- ✓ 1 cup regular flour
- ✓ 3 eggs
- ✓ 1 tablespoon dark rum
- ✓ ¼ teaspoon cinnamon powder
- ✓ 1 teaspoon vanilla extract
- ✓ 1 ½ teaspoons baking powder

Ingredients:

- ✓ 4 tablespoons Greek yogurt
- ✓ ¼ cup coconut oil
- ✓ ¼ cup olive oil
- ✓ 2 tablespoons honey
- ✓ 1 cup brown sugar
- ✓ 4 tablespoons walnuts, chopped
- ✓ ¼ teaspoon caramel sauce

Directions:

❖ Preheat oven to 350°F. In a bowl, mix the flour, cardamom cinnamon, vanilla, baking powder and salt. In another bowl, beat the eggs with the Greek yogurt using an electric mixer. Gently add the coconut and olive oil. Combine well.

❖ Toss in the rum, honey and sugar; stir to combine. Mix the wet ingredients with the dry mixture. Stir in the peaches, raisins and nuts. Pour the mixture into a greased baking dish and bake for 30-40 minutes until a knife inserted into the center of the cake comes out clean.

❖ Remove from oven and let rest for 10 minutes, then flip onto a wire rack to cool completely. Heat the caramel sauce in a skillet and pour over the cooled cake to serve.

## 103) HEARTY CHIA AND BLACKBERRY PUDDING

| **Preparation Time**: 45 minutes | **Cooking Time**: | **Servings**: 2 |
|---|---|---|

Ingredients:

- ✓ ¼ cup chia seeds
- ✓ ½ cup blackberries, fresh
- ✓ 1 teaspoon liquid sweetener 1

Ingredients:

- ✓ cup coconut and almond milk, whole and unsweetened
- ✓ 1 teaspoon vanilla extract

Directions:

❖ Take the vanilla, liquid sweetener and coconut almond milk and add to the blender. Process until thick. Add the blackberries and process until smooth.

❖ Divide the mixture between cups and chill for 30 minutes. Serve and enjoy!

## 104) DELICATE BLACKBERRY CRUMBLE

| **Preparation Time**: 10 minutes | **Cooking Time**: 45 minutes | **Servings**: 4 |
|---|---|---|

Ingredients:

- ✓ ½ cup coconut flour
- ✓ ½ cup banana, peeled and mashed
- ✓ 6 tablespoons water
- ✓ 3 cups fresh blackberries

Ingredients:

- ✓ ½ cup arrowroot flour
- ✓ 1 ½ teaspoons baking soda
- ✓ 4 tablespoons almond butter, melted
- ✓ 1 tablespoon fresh lemon juice

Directions:

❖ Preheat oven to 300 degrees F. Take a baking sheet and lightly grease it. Take a bowl and mix all ingredients except blackberries, mix well.

❖ Place the blackberries in the bottom of the baking dish and cover with flour. Bake for 40 minutes. Serve and enjoy!

## 105) AMAZING MAPLE PECAN BACON SLICES

| **Preparation Time**: 10 minutes | **Cooking Time**: 25 minutes + freezing time | **Servings**: 12 |
|---|---|---|

Ingredients:

- ✓ 1 tablespoon sugar-free maple syrup
- ✓ 12 slices of bacon
- ✓ Granular Stevia to taste
- ✓ 15-20 drops of Stevia

Ingredients:

- ✓ For the coating:
- ✓ 4 tablespoons dark cocoa powder
- ✓ ¼ cup pecans, chopped
- ✓ 15-20 drops of Stevia

Directions:

❖ Take a baking sheet and lay the bacon slices on it. Rub with maple syrup and Stevia, turn the slices over and do the same with the other side. Bake for 10-15 minutes at 220 degrees F. After baking, drain bacon grease.

❖ To form a batter, mix the bacon fat, Stevia and cocoa powder. Dip the bacon slices in the batter and roll in the chopped pecans. Allow to air dry until the chocolate hardens.

## 106) CARROT BALL DELIGHT

| **Preparation Time**: 10minutes | **Cooking Time**: | **Servings: 4** |
|---|---|---|

Ingredients:

- ✓ 6 pitted Medjool dates
- ✓ 1 carrot, finely grated
- ✓ ¼ cup raw walnuts

Ingredients:

- ✓ ¼ cup unsweetened coconut, shredded
- ✓ 1 teaspoon nutmeg
- ✓ 1/8 teaspoon sunflower seeds

Directions:

- ❖ Take a food processor and add dates, ¼ cup grated carrots, coconut sunflower seeds, nutmeg. Blend well and reduce the mixture to a puree.

- ❖ Add the nuts and the remaining ¼ cup of carrots. Pulse the mixture until chunky in consistency. Form balls with your hand and roll them in the coconut. Top with the carrots and chill. Enjoy!

## 107) SPICE FRIENDLY MUFFINS

| **Preparation Time**: 5 minutes | **Cooking Time**: 45 minutes | **Servings: 12** |
|---|---|---|

Ingredients:

- ✓ ½ cup raw hemp hearts
- ✓ ½ cup flax seeds
- ✓ ¼ cup chia seeds
- ✓ 2 tablespoons Psyllium husk powder

Ingredients:

- ✓ 1 tablespoon cinnamon stevia flavor
- ✓ ½ teaspoon baking powder
- ✓ ½ teaspoon sunflower seeds
- ✓ 1 cup water

Directions:

- ❖ preheat oven to 350 degrees F. Line muffin tray with liners. Take a large bowl and add the peanut almond butter, pumpkin, sweetener, coconut almond milk, flax seeds and mix well. Continue to mix until the mixture has been completely combined. Take another bowl and add the baking powder, spices, and coconut flour. Mix well.

- ❖ Add the dry ingredients to the wet bowl and mix until the coconut flour has mixed well. Let sit for a while until the coconut flour has absorbed all the moisture.
- ❖ Divide the mixture between your muffin pans and bake for 45 minutes. Enjoy!

## 108) FANTASTIC CAULIFLOWER BAGELS

| **Preparation Time**: 10 minutes | **Cooking Time**: 30 minutes | **Servings: 12** |
|---|---|---|

Ingredients:

- ✓ 1 large cauliflower, floreted and coarsely chopped
- ✓ ¼ cup nutritional yeast
- ✓ ¼ cup almond flour
- ✓ ½ teaspoon garlic powder

Ingredients:

- ✓ 1 ½ teaspoons fine sea sunflower seeds
- ✓ 1 whole egg
- ✓ 1 tablespoon sesame seeds

- ❖ preheat oven to 400 degrees F. Line a baking sheet with parchment paper; set aside. Blend the cauliflower in the food processor and transfer to a bowl.
- ❖ Add the nutritional yeast, almond flour, garlic powder and sunflower seeds to a bowl, mix. Take another bowl and beat the eggs, add to the cauliflower mix. Give the mixture a stir. Incorporate the dough into the egg mixture.

- ❖ Make balls with the dough, poking a hole in each ball with your thumb. Place them on the prepared sheet, flattening them into a bagel shape. Sprinkle with sesame seeds and bake for 30 minutes. Remove from oven and let them cool, enjoy!

## 109)  SAVORY LIME PIE

| **Preparation Time**: 5 minutes | **Cooking Time**: 5 minutes + freezing time | **Servings: 12** |
|---|---|---|

Ingredients:

- ✓ 1 tablespoon ground cinnamon
- ✓ 3 tablespoons almond butter
- ✓ 1 cup almond flour

  For the filling:
- ✓ 3 tablespoons grass-fed almond butter

Ingredients:

- ✓ 4 ounces whole cream cheese
- ✓ ¼ cup coconut oil
- ✓ 2 limes
- ✓ A handful of baby spinach Stevia to taste

Directions:

❖ Mix the cinnamon and almond butter to form a crumble mixture. Press this mixture into the bottom of 12 muffin cups. Bake for 7 minutes at 350 degrees F.

❖ Squeeze the lime and grate the zest while the crust is baking. Take a food processor and add all the filling ingredients. Blend until smooth. Let cool naturally. Pour the mixture into the center. Freeze until set and serve.

## 110)  THE PERFECT PONZU ORANGE

| **Preparation Time**: 30 minutes | **Cooking Time**: 5 minutes | **Servings: 8** |
|---|---|---|

Ingredients:

- ✓ ¼ cup coconut amino acids
- ✓ ½ cup rice vinegar
- ✓ 2 tablespoons dried fish flakes

Ingredients:

- ✓ 1 (1 inch) square kombu (kelp)
- ✓ 1 orange, quartered

Directions:

❖ Take a saucepan and place it over medium heat. Add the coconut amino acid, rice vinegar, fish flakes, kombu, and orange quarters and let the mixture sit for 30 minutes.

❖ Bring the mixture to a boil and immediately remove from heat. Allow to cool and strain through cheesecloth. Serve and enjoy!

## 111)  THE REFRESHING NUTTER

| **Preparation Time**: 10 minutes | **Cooking Time**: | **Servings: 1** |
|---|---|---|

Ingredients:

- ✓ 1 tablespoon chia seeds
- ✓ 2 cups water 1 ounce macadamia nuts

Ingredients:

- ✓ 1-2 packets Stevia, optional
- ✓ 1 ounce hazelnuts

Directions:

❖ Add all of the listed ingredients to a blender. Blend on high speed until smooth and creamy. Enjoy your smoothie.

| **112)** | **APPLE AND ALMOND MUFFINS** |
|---|---|

| **Preparation Time**: 10 minutes | **Cooking Time:** 20 minutes | **Servings: 6 muffins** |
|---|---|---|

Ingredients:

- ✓ 6 ounces ground almonds
- ✓ 1 teaspoon cinnamon
- ✓ ½ teaspoon baking powder
- ✓ 1 pinch sunflower seeds

Ingredients:

- ✓ 1 whole egg
- ✓ 1 teaspoon apple cider vinegar
- ✓ 2 tablespoons erythritol
- ✓ 1/3 cup applesauce

Directions:

❖ Preheat oven to 350 degrees F. Line a muffin pan with paper muffin cups; set aside. Mix the almonds, cinnamon, baking powder, and sunflower seeds together and set aside. Take another bowl and whisk eggs, apple cider vinegar, applesauce, erythritol.

❖ Add the mix to the dry ingredients and mix well until you have a smooth batter. Pour the batter into the mold and bake for 20 minutes. Once done, let them cool. Serve and enjoy!

| **113)** | **MATCHA BOMB SUPREME** |
|---|---|

| **Preparation Time**: 100 minutes | **Cooking Time:** | **Servings: 10** |
|---|---|---|

Ingredients:

- ✓ 3/4 cup hemp seeds
- ✓ ½ cup coconut oil
- ✓ 2 tablespoons coconut almond butter
- ✓ 1 teaspoon Matcha powder

Ingredients:

- ✓ 2 tablespoons vanilla bean extract
- ✓ ½ teaspoon mint extract
- ✓ Liquid stevia

Directions:

❖ Take your blender/ food processor and add the hemp seeds, coconut oil, Matcha, vanilla extract and stevia.

❖ Blend until you have a nice batter and divide into silicone molds. Melt the coconut and almond butter and pour over top. Let the cups cool and enjoy!

| **114)** | **PINEAPPLE HEARTY PUDDING** |
|---|---|

| **Preparation Time**: 10 minutes | **Cooking Time:** 5 hours | **Servings: 4** |
|---|---|---|

Ingredients:

- ✓ 1 teaspoon baking powder
- ✓ 1 cup coconut flour
- ✓ 3 tablespoons stevia
- ✓ 3 tablespoons avocado oil
- ✓ ½ cup coconut milk

Ingredients:

- ✓ ½ cup pecans, chopped
- ✓ ½ cup pineapple, chopped
- ✓ ½ cup lemon zest, grated
- ✓ 1 cup pineapple juice, natural

Directions:

❖ Grease the Slow Cooker with oil. Take a bowl and mix the flour, stevia, baking powder, oil, milk, pecans, pineapple, lemon zest, pineapple juice and mix well.

❖ Pour the mixture into the slow stove. Put the lid on and cook on LOW for 5 hours. Divide between bowls and serve. Enjoy!

## 115) TASTY POACHED APPLES

| **Preparation Time**: 10 minutes | **Cooking Time:** 2 hours 30 minutes | **Servings:** 8 |
|---|---|---|

| Ingredients: | Ingredients: |
|---|---|
| ✓ 6 apples, cored, peeled and sliced<br>✓ 1 cup apple juice, natural | ✓ 1 cup coconut sugar<br>✓ 1 tablespoon cinnamon powder |
| Directions:<br><br>❖ Grease the Slow Cooker with cooking spray. Add the apples, sugar, juice and cinnamon to the slow stove. Stir gently. | ❖ Put the lid on and cook on HIGH for 4 hours. Serve cold and enjoy! |

## 116) HEART-WARMING CINNAMON RICE PUDDING

| **Preparation Time**: 10 minutes | **Cooking Time:** 5 hours | **Servings:** 4 |
|---|---|---|

| Ingredients: | Ingredients: |
|---|---|
| ✓ 6 ½ cups water<br>✓ 1 cup coconut sugar<br>✓ 2 cups white rice | ✓ 2 cinnamon sticks<br>✓ ½ cup coconut, shredded |
| Directions:<br><br>❖ Add the water, rice, sugar, cinnamon and coconut to your Slow Cooker. Stir gently. Put the lid on and cook on HIGH for 5 hours. Discard the cinnamon. | ❖ Divide the pudding between dessert plates and enjoy! |

## 117) SWEET ALMOND AND COCONUT FAT BOMBS

| **Preparation Time**: 10 minutes | **Cooking Time:** MOU4]<br>Freezing Time: + 20 minutes | **Servings:** 6 |
|---|---|---|

| Ingredients: | Ingredients: |
|---|---|
| ✓ ¼ cup melted coconut oil<br>✓ 9 ½ tablespoons almond butter<br>✓ 90 drops liquid stevia | ✓ 3 tablespoons cocoa<br>✓ 9 tablespoons melted almond butter sunflower seeds |
| Directions:<br><br>❖ Take a bowl and add all the ingredients listed. Mix them together well. Pour 2 tablespoons of the mixture into as many muffin molds as you want. | ❖ Chill for 20 minutes and take them out. Serve and enjoy! |

## 118)  THE MOST ELEGANT PARSLEY SOUFFLÉ EVER

| Preparation Time: 5 minutes | Cooking Time: 6 minutes | Servings: 5 |
|---|---|---|

| | |
|---|---|
| ✓ 2 whole eggs<br>✓ 1 fresh red pepper, chopped | ✓ 2 tablespoons coconut cream<br>✓ 1 tablespoon fresh parsley, chopped<br>Sunflower seeds to taste |
| ❖ Preheat oven to 390 degrees F. Butter almonds in 2 souffle dishes. Add ingredients to a blender and mix well. Divide the batter among the soufflé dishes and bake for 6 minutes. Serve and enjoy! | |

## 119)  EXUBERANT COCONUT CARAMEL

| Preparation Time: 20 minutes | Cooking Time: 2 hours | Servings: 12 |
|---|---|---|

| | |
|---|---|
| Ingredients:<br><br>✓ ¼ cup coconut, shredded<br>✓ 2 cups coconut oil<br>✓ ½ cup coconut cream<br>✓ ¼ cup almonds, shredded | Ingredients:<br><br>✓ 1 teaspoon almond extract<br>✓ A pinch of sunflower seeds<br>✓ Stevia to taste |
| ❖ Take a large bowl and pour in the coconut cream and coconut oil. Whisk with an electric beater. Whisk until the mixture becomes smooth and glossy | ❖ Add the cocoa powder slowly and mix well. Add the rest of the ingredients. Pour into a loaf pan lined with baking paper. Freeze until firm. Cut into squares and serve. |

## 120)  PUMPKIN PUDDING WITH CHIA SEEDS EASY

| Preparation Time: 10-15 minutes | Cooking Time: | Servings: 4 |
|---|---|---|

| | |
|---|---|
| Ingredients:<br><br>✓ 1 cup maple syrup<br>✓ 2 teaspoons pumpkin spice<br>✓ 1 cup pumpkin puree | Ingredients:<br><br>✓ 1 ¼ cup almond milk<br>✓ ½ cup chia seeds |
| ❖ Add all ingredients to a bowl and mix gently. Leave in the refrigerator overnight or at least 15 minutes. Add desired ingredients such as blueberries, almonds, etc. Serve and enjoy! | |

## 121)  DECISIVE LIME AND STRAWBERRY POPSICLE

| Preparation Time: 2 hours | Cooking Time: | Servings: 4 |
|---|---|---|

| | |
|---|---|
| Ingredients:<br><br>✓ 1 tablespoon lime juice, fresh<br>✓ ¼ cup strawberries, hulled and sliced | Ingredients:<br><br>✓ ¼ cup coconut almond milk, unsweetened and full-fat<br>✓ 2 teaspoons natural sweetener |
| ❖ Blend the listed ingredients in a blender until smooth. Pour mixture into popsicle molds and let cool for 2 hours. Serve and enjoy! | |

| 122) | COCONUT BREAD | |
|---|---|---|
| **Preparation Time**: 15 minutes | **Cooking Time:** 40 minutes | **Servings: 4** |

Ingredients:

- ✓ 1 ½ tablespoons coconut flour
- ✓ ¼ teaspoon baking powder
- ✓ 1/8 teaspoon sunflower seeds

Ingredients:

- ✓ 1 tablespoon coconut oil, melted
- ✓ 1 whole egg

Directions:

❖ Preheat the oven to 350 degrees F. Add the coconut flour, baking powder, and sunflower seeds. Add the coconut oil, eggs and mix well until combined.

❖ Allow the batter to sit for a few minutes. Pour half of the batter onto the baking sheet. Spread to form a circle, repeat with remaining batter. Bake in the oven for 10 minutes. Once golden brown, let cool and serve. Enjoy!

| 123) | AUTHENTIC MEDJOOL DATE TRUFFLES | |
|---|---|---|
| **Preparation Time**: 10-15 minutes | **Cooking Time:** | **Servings: 4** |

Ingredients:

- ✓ 2 tablespoons peanut oil
- ✓ ½ cup popcorn kernels
- ✓ 1/3 cup peanuts, chopped

Ingredients:

- ✓ 1/3 cup almond and peanut butter
- ✓ ¼ cup wildflower honey

Directions:

❖ Take a pot and add the popcorn kernels, peanut oil. Put it on medium heat and shake the pot gently until all the corn has popped.

❖ Take a saucepan and add the honey, simmer gently for 2-3 minutes. Add the almond and peanut butter and stir. Coat the popcorn with the mixture and enjoy!

| 124) | JUST A MINUTE THAT'S WORTH A MUFFIN | |
|---|---|---|
| **Preparation Time**: 5 minutes | **Cooking Time:** 1 minute | **Servings: 2** |

Ingredients:

- ✓ Coconut oil for greasing
- ✓ 2 teaspoons coconut flour
- ✓ 1 pinch baking soda

Ingredients:

- ✓ 1 pinch sunflower seeds
- ✓ 1 whole egg

Directions:

❖ Grease the ramekin with coconut oil and set aside. Add ingredients to a bowl and combine until there are no lumps. Pour the batter into the ramekin. Microwave for 1 minute on HIGH. Cut in half and serve. Enjoy!

| 125) | POACHED PEARS IN RED WINE | |
|---|---|---|
| **Preparation Time**: 1 hour 35 minutes | **Cooking Time:** | **Servings: 4** |

**Ingredients:**

- ✓ 4 pears, peeled with stem intact
- ✓ 2 cups red wine
- ✓ 8 whole cloves
- ✓ 1 cinnamon stick

**Ingredients:**

- ✓ ½ teaspoon vanilla extract
- ✓ 2 teaspoons sugar
- ✓ Creme fraiche for garnish

**Directions:**

- ❖ In a saucepan over low heat, mix the red wine, cinnamon stick, cloves, vanilla extract and sugar and bring to a boil, stirring often until the sugar is dissolved. Add the pears, making sure they are submerged and boil for 15-20 minutes.

- ❖ Remove the pears to a plate and let the liquid simmer over medium heat for 15 minutes until reduced by half and syrupy. Remove from heat and let cool for 10 minutes. Drain to discard spices, allow to cool and pour over pears. Add the creme fraiche and serve.

| 126) | SICILIAN GRANITA | |
|---|---|---|
| **Preparation Time**: 5 minutes + freezing tme | **Cooking Time:** | **Servings: 4** |

**Ingredients:**

- ✓ 4 small oranges, chopped
- ✓ ½ teaspoon almond extract
- ✓ 2 tablespoons lemon juice

**Ingredients:**

- ✓ 1 cup orange juice
- ✓ ¼ cup honey
- ✓ Fresh mint leaves for garnish

**Directions:**

- ❖ In a food processor, blend the oranges, orange juice, honey, almond extract and lemon juice. Pulse until smooth. Pour into a dipping dish and freeze for 1 hour.

- ❖ Stir with a fork and freeze for another 30 minutes. Repeat a couple of times. Pour into dessert glasses and garnish with basil leaves. Serve immediately.

| 127) | FRUIT CUPS WITH ORANGE JUICE | |
|---|---|---|
| **Preparation Time**: 10 minutes | **Cooking Time:** | **Servings: 4** |

**Ingredients:**

- ✓ 1 cup orange juice
- ✓ ½ cup watermelon cubes
- ✓ 1 ½ cups grapes, cut in half
- ✓ 1 cup chopped melon

**Ingredients:**

- ✓ ½ cup cherries, pitted and chopped
- ✓ 1 peach, chopped
- ✓ ½ teaspoon cinnamon powder

**Directions:**

- ❖ Combine the watermelon cubes, grapes, cherries, cantaloupe and peach in a bowl. Add the orange juice and mix well. Distribute into dessert cups, sprinkle with cinnamon and serve cold.

# BOOK 2: "THE DASH DIET Cookbook"

# Chapter 1.
# BREAKFAST AND SNACKS

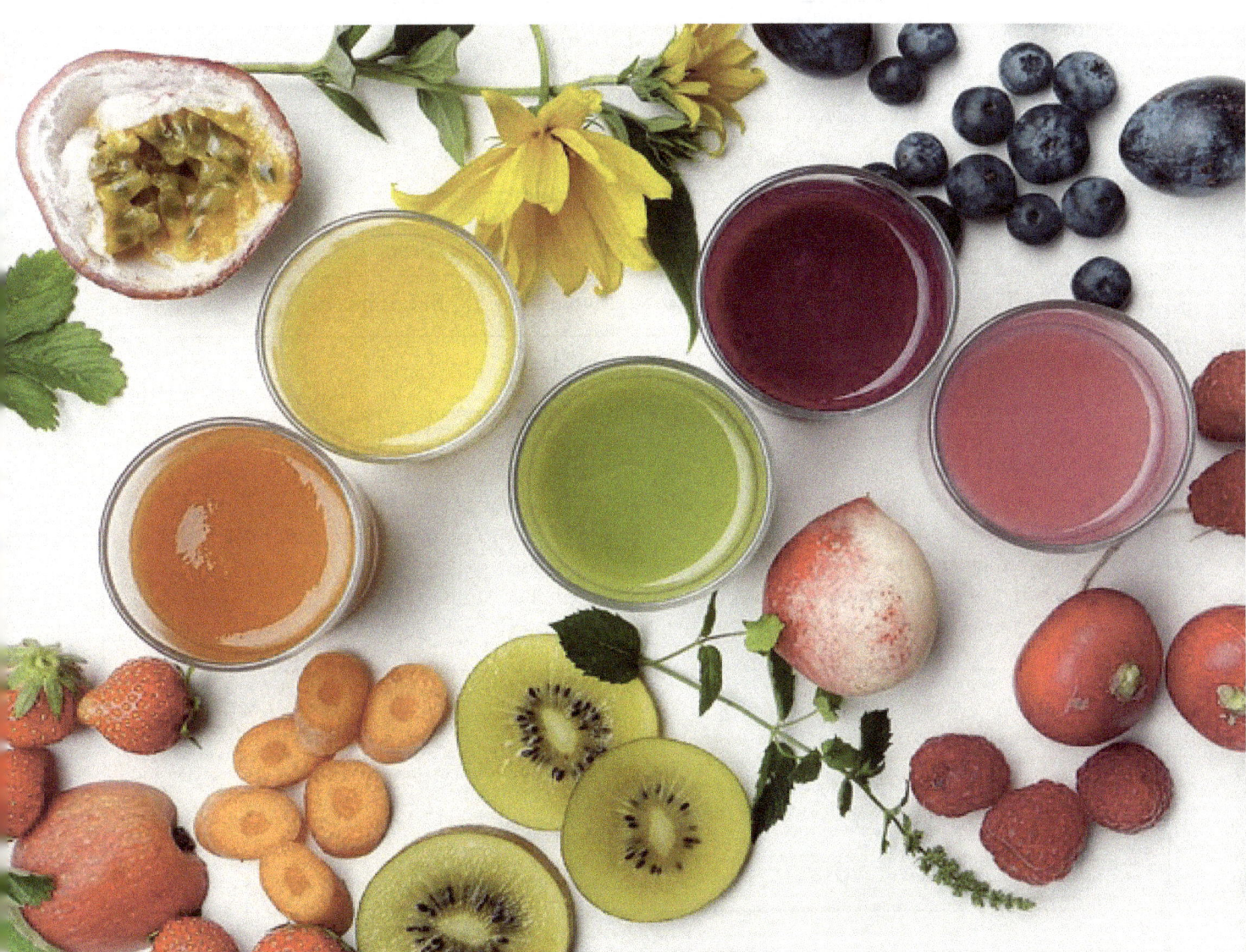

| 128) | OATMEAL COOKIES WITH MIXED NUTS | |
|---|---|---|
| **Preparation Time**: 10 minutes | **Cooking Time**: 12 minutes | **Servings: 40 cookies** |

Ingredients:

- ✓ 1⅓ cups of uncooked old oats or quick-cooking rolled oats
- ✓ 1 cup whole wheat flour
- ✓ 1 teaspoon baking powder
- ✓ 1 teaspoon ground cinnamon
- ✓ ¼ teaspoon of ground mace
- ✓ ½ cup of melted brown sugar
- ✓ ⅓ cup of plain low-fat yogurt

Ingredients:

- ✓ 2 tablespoons of canola oil
- ✓ 1 egg
- ✓ 1 teaspoon of vanilla extract
- ✓ ½ cup mixed nuts
- ✓ ½ cup of dark chocolate chips

Directions:

- ❖ Preheat oven to 350ºF (180ºC). Line two baking sheets with baking mats or parchment paper.
- ❖ In a medium bowl, mix together oats, flour, baking powder, cinnamon, mace and sugar.
- ❖ In a large bowl, mix together yogurt, oil, egg and vanilla. Add the flour mixture to the yogurt mixture.

- ❖ Using a spatula, mix until just combined. Stir in the dried fruit and chocolate chips.
- ❖ Using a spoon, drop the cookie dough onto a baking sheet about 2 inches apart.
- ❖ Bake 10 to 12 minutes, until lightly browned. Remove from oven and cool on a wire rack.

| 129) | APPLE PIE WITH CINNAMON SUGAR | |
|---|---|---|
| **Preparation Time**: 15 minutes | **Cooking Time**: 20 minutes | **Servings: 16** |

Ingredients:

- ✓ 1¾ cups granulated sugar
- ✓ 3 teaspoons ground cinnamon
- ✓ 1½ cups all-purpose flour
- ✓ 1½ teaspoon baking powder
- ✓ ½ teaspoon ground ginger
- ✓ ¼ teaspoon ground nutmeg
- ✓ ¼ teaspoon of ground mace
- ✓ ½ cup (4 ounces / 113 g) of low-fat cream cheese

Ingredients:

- ✓ ⅓ cup unsweetened applesauce
- ✓ 2 tablespoons of canola oil
- ✓ 1 teaspoon of vanilla extract
- ✓ 2 egg whites
- ✓ 3 Fuji apples, peeled and cut into 1 inch pieces
- ✓ Kitchen spray

Directions:

- ❖ Preheat the oven to 350ºF (180ºC). Spray one 8-inch springform or four mini springforms with cooking spray.
- ❖ In a small bowl, mix ¼ cup sugar with 2 teaspoons cinnamon. Set aside.
- ❖ In a medium bowl, combine the flour, baking powder, ginger, nutmeg, mace and remaining teaspoon of cinnamon. Set aside.
- ❖ In the bowl of a stand mixer fitted with the paddle attachment, beat 1 1/2 cups of the sugar, cream cheese, applesauce, canola oil, and vanilla extract until well blended, about 4 minutes.

- ❖ Add the egg whites to the batter and continue beating until incorporated. Add the flour mixture to the batter, ¼ cup at a time, mixing until well incorporated.
- ❖ In another small bowl, mix the apples with 3 tablespoons of the sugar and cinnamon mixture. Gently stir the apple and cinnamon mixture into the batter.
- ❖ Pour the batter into the baking dish(s) and sprinkle with the remaining cinnamon sugar.
- ❖ Bake for 20 minutes, or until a toothpick inserted into the center comes out clean. Individual pans will bake more quickly; check after 12 minutes.

## 130)   GRILLED PRUNES WITH HONEY AND CINNAMON

| **Preparation Time**: 10 minutes | **Cooking Time**: 15 minutes | **Servings: 4** |
|---|---|---|

Ingredients:

- ✓ 4 large plums, cut in half and pitted
- ✓ 1 tablespoon of olive oil
- ✓ 1 tablespoon of honey

Ingredients:

- ✓ 1 teaspoon ground cinnamon
- ✓ 2 cups of vanilla frozen yogurt

Directions:

- ❖ Preheat grill to medium heat.
- ❖ Brush the plum halves with olive oil. Grill, flesh side down, for 4 to 5 minutes, then flip and cook for another 4 to 5 minutes, until tender.

- ❖ In a small bowl, whisk together the honey and cinnamon.
- ❖ Distribute frozen yogurt among 4 bowls. Place 2 plum halves in each bowl and drizzle each with the cinnamon and honey mixture.

## 131)   CHOCOLATE COOKIES WITH PEANUT BUTTER AND OATMEAL

| **Preparation Time**: 15 minutes | **Cooking Time**: 10 minutes | **Servings: 24 cookies** |
|---|---|---|

Ingredients:

- ✓ 1½ cups creamy natural peanut butter
- ✓ ½ cup dark brown sugar
- ✓ 2 big eggs
- ✓ 1 cup old-fashioned rolled oats

Ingredients:

- ✓ 1 teaspoon of baking soda
- ✓ ½ teaspoon of kosher salt or sea salt
- ✓ ½ cup of dark chocolate chips

Directions:

- ❖ Preheat the oven to 350°F (180°C). Line a baking sheet with baking paper.
- ❖ In the bowl of a mixer fitted with the paddle attachment, beat the peanut butter until very smooth. Continue beating and add the brown sugar, then one egg at a time, until frothy. Beat in the oats, baking soda and salt until combined. Add in the dark chocolate chips.

- ❖ Use a small cookie scoop or teaspoon and place balls of cookie dough on the baking sheet, about 2 inches apart. Bake for 8-10 minutes, depending on your preferred baking level.

## 132)    PEACH CRUMBLE MUFFINS

| **Preparation Time**: 25 minutes | **Cooking Time**: 25 minutes | **Servings: 12 muffins** |
|---|---|---|

Ingredients:

Crumble:
- ✓ 2 tablespoons of dark brown sugar
- ✓ 1 tablespoon of honey
- ✓ 1 teaspoon ground cinnamon
- ✓ 2 tablespoons of canola oil
- ✓ ½ cup rolled old oats

Peach Muffins:
- ✓ 1¾ cups whole wheat flour or whole wheat pasta flour
- ✓ 1 teaspoon baking powder
- ✓ 1 teaspoon of baking soda

Ingredients:
- ✓ 1 teaspoon ground cinnamon
- ✓ ½ teaspoon ground ginger
- ✓ ½ teaspoon of kosher salt or sea salt
- ✓ ¼ cup canola oil
- ✓ ¼ cup dark brown sugar
- ✓ 2 big eggs
- ✓ 1½ teaspoons of vanilla extract
- ✓ ¼ cup of fat-free Greek yogurt
- ✓ 3 peaches, diced (about 1 1/2 cups)

Directions:

- ❖ Preheat the oven to 425ºF (220ºC). Line a 12-cup muffin mold with muffin liners and spray with cooking spray.
- ❖ Making the crumble
- ❖ In a small bowl, mix together brown sugar, honey, cinnamon, canola oil and oats until combined. Set aside.
- ❖ Making muffins
- ❖ In a large bowl, whisk together the flour, baking powder, baking soda, cinnamon, ginger and salt.

- ❖ In another bowl, use a hand mixer to beat together the canola oil, brown sugar, and one egg at a time until frothy. Add the vanilla extract and yogurt. Slowly add the flour mixture to the bowl and beat until the ingredients are just combined. Add the diced peaches with a spatula.
- ❖ Fill each muffin about three-quarters full with the batter. Spoon the crumble mixture on top of each muffin. Bake for 5-6 minutes, then reduce the oven temperature to 350ºF (180ºC) and bake for another 15-18 minutes, until a toothpick inserted in the center comes out clean. Let cool slightly before removing from muffin pan.
- ❖ Once completely cooled, store in a sealed plastic bag in the refrigerator for up to 5 days or freeze for up to 2 months.

## 133)    BAKED APPLES WITH CINNAMON AND WALNUTS

| **Preparation Time**: 10 minutes | **Cooking Time**: 25 minutes | **Servings: 4** |
|---|---|---|

Ingredients:

- ✓ 4 hard-boiled apples, such as Cortland or Granny Smith, peeled and cored
- ✓ 3 teaspoons of light brown sugar
- ✓ ½ teaspoon of cinnamon
- ✓ ½ teaspoon of cardamom
- ✓ 1 cup unsweetened apple cider

Ingredients:

- ✓ 1 cup unsweetened orange juice
- ✓ 1 tablespoon of cornstarch
- ✓ 2 tablespoons of cold water
- ✓ 2 tablespoons of chopped black walnuts

Directions:

- ❖ Preheat the oven to 350ºF (180ºC).
- ❖ Place apples in a lined baking dish and sprinkle with brown sugar, cinnamon and cardamom.
- ❖ Pour the cider and orange juice into the dish and bake for 20-25 minutes. Remove apples to 4 dessert plates and set aside.

- ❖ Pour the cooking juices into a small saucepan and heat over medium heat until simmering. In a separate bowl, mix the cornstarch and water, then whisk into the saucepan. Continue stirring until thickened, then spoon over each apple. Sprinkle chopped walnuts over each serving and serve warm.

## 134) RASPBERRY AND WALNUT SORBET

| **Preparation Time**: 5 minutes | **Cooking Time**: 0 minutes | **Servings: 5** |
|---|---|---|

Ingredients:

- ✓ 2 cups of fresh ripe raspberries
- ✓ ¼ cup chopped walnuts

Ingredients:

- ✓ 1 teaspoon of lemon juice
- ✓ 2 tablespoons of organic agave nectar

Directions:

- ❖ In a food processor or blender, puree all ingredients. Freeze in an ice cream maker. Alternatively, spread the fruit mixture on a cookie sheet and place in the freezer.

- ❖ Every 20 minutes, scrape the fruit mixture with a spoon so it doesn't freeze into a solid mass (this will keep it nice and light).

## 135) VANILLA PUMPKIN PUDDING

| **Preparation Time**: 5 minutes | **Cooking Time**: 0 minutes | **Servings: 6** |
|---|---|---|

Ingredients:

- ✓ 1½ cups non-fat vanilla yogurt
- ✓ 1 (20-ounce / 567-g) can of plain pumpkin puree
- ✓ ½ teaspoon ground nutmeg

Ingredients:

- ✓ ½ teaspoon ground cinnamon
- ✓ 1 vanilla pod

Directions:

- ❖ Combine the yogurt, pumpkin puree, nutmeg and cinnamon in a medium sized bowl. Scrape the vanilla seeds from the peel and place in the mixture.

- ❖ Mix well until all ingredients are combined. Chill until ready to serve.

## 136) CHOCOLATE MERINGUE PUFFS

| **Preparation Time**: 5 minutes | **Cooking Time**: 12 minutes | **Servings: 3 Dozens** |
|---|---|---|

Ingredients:

- ✓ 3 medium egg whites
- ✓ ½ teaspoon of cream of tartar
- ✓ ½ cup of sugar
- ✓ ½ teaspoon of orange extract

Ingredients:

- ✓ 1½ tablespoons of cocoa powder
- ✓ 6 ounces (170 g) bittersweet chocolate, melted but not hot
- ✓ Olive oil cooking spray

Directions:

- ❖ Preheat the oven to 350°F (180°C).
- ❖ In a dry medium-sized glass bowl, beat egg whites and cream of tartar with a hand mixer on medium speed until peaks begin to form, about 1 minute. Add the sugar slowly while continuing to mix.
- ❖ Add the orange extract and continue beating, scraping the sides of the bowl often, until the mixture forms firm peaks and is glossy.

- ❖ In a separate bowl, mix the cocoa with the melted chocolate, then gently add the mixture to the meringue. Line baking sheets with parchment paper, then apply olive oil cooking spray. Drop rounded tablespoons of mixture onto the baking paper.
- ❖ Bake on the middle rack for 8-12 minutes until the puffs are firm on the outside but still soft on the inside. You may want to switch to the top rack for the last couple of minutes so that the bottoms don't darken. When the puffs are cool, remove them from the parchment paper and store in an airtight container for up to 1 week.

## 137)  BREAKFAST QUESADILLAS WITH BLACK BEANS

| **Preparation Time**: 15 minutes | **Cooking Time:** 15 minutes | **Servings: 2** |
| --- | --- | --- |

Ingredients:

- ✓  2 eggs
- ✓  2 egg whites
- ✓  2 to 4 tablespoons of skim or low-fat milk
- ✓  ¼ teaspoon freshly ground black pepper
- ✓  1 large tomato, chopped
- ✓  2 tablespoons of chopped coriander

Ingredients:

- ✓  ½ cup canned black beans, rinsed and drained
- ✓  1½ tablespoons olive oil, divided
- ✓  4 corn tortillas
- ✓  ½ avocado, peeled, pitted and cut into thin slices

Directions:

- ❖  In a bowl, combine the eggs, egg whites, milk and black pepper. Using an electric mixer, beat until smooth. In the same bowl, add the tomato, cilantro and black beans and incorporate them into the eggs with a spoon.
- ❖  Heat half of the olive oil in a medium skillet over medium heat. Add the scrambled egg mixture and cook for a few minutes, stirring, until cooked through. Remove from skillet.

- ❖  Divide the scrambled egg mixture among the tortillas, layering only on one half of the tortilla.
- ❖  Top with avocado slices and fold tortillas in half.
- ❖  Heat the remaining oil over medium heat and add one of the folded tortillas to the pan. Cook for 1 to 2 minutes on each side, or until golden brown. Repeat with the remaining tortillas.
- ❖  Serve immediately.

## 138)  BREAKFAST WITH STUFFED PEPPERS

| **Preparation Time**: 5 minutes | **Cooking Time:** 35 to 45 minutes | **Servings: 4** |
| --- | --- | --- |

Ingredients:

- ✓  4 peppers (any color)
- ✓  1 (16-ounce / 454-g) bag of frozen spinach
- ✓  4 eggs

Ingredients:

- ✓  ¼ cup shredded low-fat cheese (optional)
- ✓  Freshly ground black pepper to taste

Directions:

- ❖  Preheat the oven to 400ºF (205ºC). Line a baking sheet with aluminum foil.
- ❖  Cut the tops off each bell pepper and remove the seeds. Discard the tops and seeds.
- ❖  Place the peppers in the baking dish and bake for about 15 minutes.
- ❖  While the peppers are cooking, thaw the spinach and drain off any excess moisture.

- ❖  Remove peppers from oven and fill bottom evenly with thawed spinach.
- ❖  Crack an egg on top of the spinach inside each bell pepper. Top each egg with a tablespoon of cheese (if using) and season with black pepper, to taste.
- ❖  Bake for about 15-20 minutes, or until egg whites are set and opaque.

| 139) | BREAKFAST RICE PORRIDGE WITH APRICOTS | |
|---|---|---|
| **Preparation Time**: 2 minutes | **Cooking Time:** 8 minutes | **Servings: 4** |

Ingredients:

- ✓ 3 cups of cooked brown rice
- ✓ 1¾ cups of skim or low-fat milk
- ✓ 2 tablespoons lightly packed brown sugar
- ✓ 4 dried apricots, chopped

Ingredients:

- ✓ 1 medium apple, cored and diced
- ✓ ¾ teaspoon ground cinnamon
- ✓ ¾ teaspoon of vanilla extract

Directions:

❖ In a medium saucepan, combine the rice, milk, sugar, apricots, apple and cinnamon. Bring to a boil over medium heat, then lower heat slightly and cook, stirring often, for 2 to 3 minutes or until porridge reaches desired thickness.

❖ Turn off the heat and stir in the vanilla extract.

❖ Serve hot.

# Chapter 2.  LUNCH

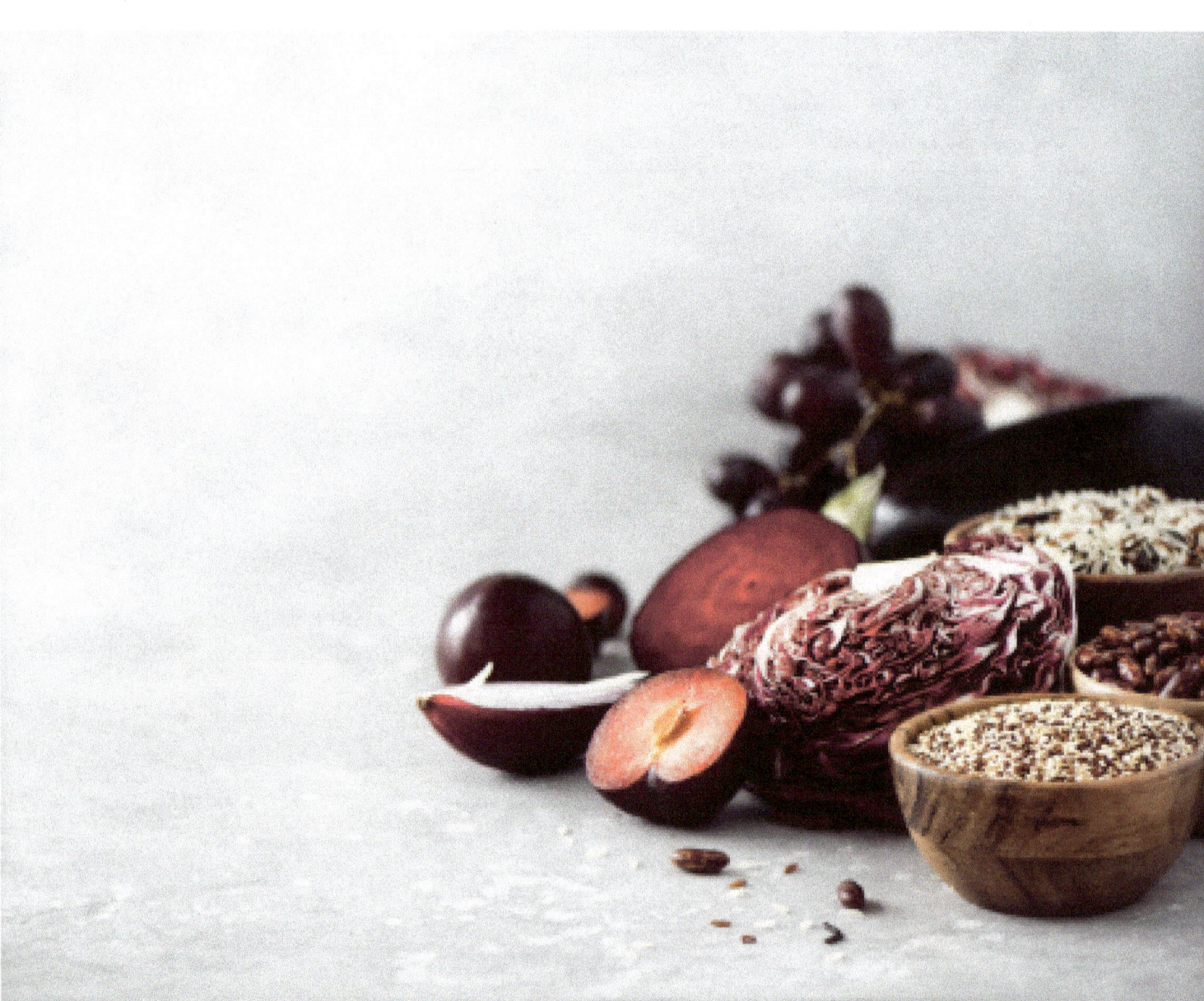

| *140)* | **CURRIED RED LENTILS** | |
|---|---|---|
| **Preparation Time**: 15 minutes | **Cooking Time**: 23 minutes | **Servings**: 8 |

Ingredients:

- ✓ 2 cups red lentils, rinsed
- ✓ 1 tablespoon extra virgin olive oil
- ✓ 1 large onion, chopped
- ✓ 1 teaspoon fresh ginger, chopped
- ✓ 1 teaspoon garlic, minced

Ingredients:

- ✓ 2 tablespoons curry paste
- ✓ 1 tablespoon curry powder
- ✓ 1 teaspoon ground cumin
- ✓ 1 teaspoon ground turmeric
- ✓ 1 teaspoon red chili powder - Salt and freshly ground black pepper, to taste
- ✓ 1 (14¼-ounce) can be tomato puree

Directions:

- ❖ In a substantial pot of water, add the lentils and bring to a boil over high heat. Reduce heat to medium-low and simmer, covered, for about 15-20 minutes. Drain well. Meanwhile in a large skillet, heat the oil over medium heat.
- ❖ Add the onion and sauté for about twenty minutes. Meanwhile in a very bowl, mix all the remaining ingredients except the tomato puree.

- ❖ Add the spice mixture to the pan with the onions over medium-high heat. Sauté for about 1-2 minutes. Add tomato puree and cook for about 1 minute. Transfer a combination to the pan with the lentils and stir to combine. Serve hot.

| *141)* | **QUINOA WITH ASPARAGUS** | |
|---|---|---|
| **Preparation Time**: 15 minutes | **Cooking Time**: 18 minutes | **Servings**: 4 |

Ingredients:

- ✓ 1 pound fresh asparagus, chopped
- ✓ 2 teaspoons coconut oil
- ✓ ½ onion, chopped
- ✓ 2 cloves garlic, chopped

Ingredients:

- ✓ 1 cup cooked red quinoa
- ✓ 1 tablespoon turmeric powder
- ✓ ½ cup low-sodium vegetable broth
- ✓ ½ cup nutritional yeast - 1 tablespoon fresh lemon juice

Directions:

- ❖ In a large pot of boiling water, cook the asparagus for about 2-3 minutes. Drain well and rinse under cold water. In a large skillet, melt the coconut oil over medium heat.

- ❖ Add the onion and garlic and sauté for about 5 minutes. Add the quinoa, turmeric and broth and cook for about 5-6 minutes. Add the nutritional yeast, fresh lemon juice and asparagus and cook for about 3-4 minutes.

| 142) BROWN RICE CASSEROLE | | |
|---|---|---|
| **Preparation Time**: 15 minutes | **Cooking Time:** 60 minutes | **Servings: 2** |

Ingredients:

- ✓ 1 teaspoon extra-virgin olive oil
- ✓ 1 red onion, thinly sliced
- ✓ 1½ teaspoons turmeric powder
- ✓ 9 ounces brown mushrooms, sliced
- ✓ 1 teaspoon raisins

Ingredients:

- ✓ ½ cup brown rice, rinsed
- ✓ 1¼ cups vegetable broth
- ✓ ¼ cup fresh cilantro, chopped
- ✓ ½ tablespoon pine nuts, toasted
- ✓ 1 tablespoon fresh lemon juice - Salt and freshly ground black pepper, to taste

Directions:

❖ Preheat the oven to 400 degrees F. In an ovenproof casserole dish, heat the oil over medium heatAdd the onion and turmeric and sauté for about 3 minutes.

❖ Add the mushrooms and sauté about 2 minutes. Stir in the raisins, rice and broth and transfer to oven.Bake for about 45-55 minutes or until desired doneness. Just before serving, stir in remaining ingredients.

| 143) MANGO SALAD | | |
|---|---|---|
| **Preparation Time**: 15 minutes | **Cooking Time:** | **Servings: 6** |

Ingredients:

- ✓ 1 fresh Serrano pepper, chopped
- ✓ 1 tablespoon fresh cilantro, chopped
- ✓ 1 teaspoon fresh ginger, chopped
- ✓ ¼ cup golden raisins, soaked in boiling water about half an hour and drained

Ingredients:

- ✓ 3 tablespoons organic extra virgin olive oil
- ✓ 2 tablespoons balsamic vinegar - Salt, to taste
- ✓ 8 cups fresh mixed greens
- ✓ 1 medium red bell pepper, seeded and thinly sliced
- ✓ 1 large mango, peeled, pitted and diced

Directions:

❖ For the dressing in a very blender, add all ingredients and pulse until smooth. Reserve 1 tablespoon of the dressing. In a large bowl, squeeze the greens and remaining dressing and toss to coat well.

❖ In another bowl, add the bell bell pepper, mango and reserved dressing and toss to coat. Divide the greens and mango mixture among serving bowls. Serve immediately

| 144) | WHEAT BERRY AND MANGO SALAD | |
|---|---|---|
| **Preparation Time**: 20 minutes | **Cooking Time**: 35 minutes | **Servings**: 4 |

Ingredients:

- ✓ 2 cups water
- ✓ 1 cup wheat berries
- ✓ 1 mango, peeled, pitted and diced
- ✓ ½ cup red bell bell pepper, seeded and chopped
- ✓ 2 shallots, chopped
- ✓ ½ cup fresh mint leaves, chopped

Ingredients:

- ✓ ½ cup cranberries
- ✓ ½ cup walnuts, toasted and chopped
- ✓ For the dressing:
- ✓ 1 tablespoon fresh ginger, chopped - cup plain Greek yogurt
- ✓ 3 tablespoons raw honey
- ✓ ½ teaspoon balsamic vinegar - salt and freshly ground black pepper, to taste

Directions:

❖ In a saucepan, add the water and heat berries and bring to a boil. Cover and cook about 35 minutes. Remove from heat while set aside to cool. In a large bowl, add the wheat berries and remaining ingredients and stir.

❖ In a small bowl, add the dressing ingredients and beat well. Place dressing over fruit mixture and toss to coat well. Serve immediately.

| 145) | CARROT AND ALMOND SALAD | |
|---|---|---|
| **Preparation Time**: 15 minutes | **Cooking Time**: | **Servings**: 4 |

Ingredients:

- ✓ 1 garlic clove, minced –
- ✓ 2 teaspoons fresh ginger, finely grated –
- ✓ ¼ cup coconut milk
- ✓ 2 tablespoons almond butter

Ingredients:

- ✓ 2 tablespoons coconut aminos
- ✓ 1 tablespoon fresh lemon juice - pinch of cayenne - salt, to taste –
- ✓ 5 large carrots, peeled and grated - ground almonds, to taste

Directions:

❖ In a large bowl, add all ingredients except carrots and almonds and stir until well combined. Add carrots and stir to combine. Serve with the almond garnish.

| 146) | VEGETABLE AND SEED SALAD | |
|---|---|---|
| **Preparation Time**: 20 minutes | **Cooking Time:** 6 minutes | **Servings: 4** |

Ingredients:

- ✓ 1½ teaspoons fresh ginger, finely grated
- ✓ 2 tablespoons apple cider vinegar treatment
- ✓ 3 tablespoons olive oil
- ✓ 1 teaspoon sesame oil, toasted
- ✓ 3 teaspoons raw honey, divided
- ✓ ½ teaspoon red pepper flakes, crushed and divided - Salt, to taste

Ingredients:

- ✓ 1 tablespoon water
- ✓ 2 tablespoons raw sunflower seeds
- ✓ 1 tablespoon raw sesame seeds
- ✓ 1 tablespoon raw pumpkin seeds
- ✓ 10-ounce collard greens, stems and ribs removed and leaves cut thinly

Directions:

❖ For the dressing inside a bowl, add the ginger, vinegar, both oils, 1 teaspoon honey, ¼ teaspoon red pepper flakes and salt and beat until well combined.

❖ Keep aside. In another bowl, add remaining honey, remaining red pepper flakes and water and mix until well combined. Heat a medium nonstick skillet over medium heat. Add all the seeds and cook, stirring for about 3 minutes..

❖ Transfer seed mixture to a parchment paper and set aside to cool completely. Break the seed mixture into small pieces. In a large bowl, add the vegetables, 2 teaspoons with the seasoning plus a little salt and stir to coat well.

❖ Using both hands, rub the vegetables together for a few seconds. Add the remaining dressing and toss to coat well. Serve with a garnish of seed pieces. Stir in the honey mixture and cook, stirring constantly for about 3 minutes

| 147) | CABBAGE, CARROT AND RADISH SALAD | |
|---|---|---|
| **Preparation Time**: 10 minutes | **Cooking Time:** | **Servings: 4** |

Ingredients:

- ✓ 1 bunch fresh cabbage, trimmed and thinly sliced
- ✓ 1 large garlic herb, chopped
- ✓ 2 tablespoons coconut aminos
- ✓ 2 tablespoons fresh lemon juice
- ✓ 1 tablespoon organic extra virgin olive oil
- ✓ 2 tablespoons extra virgin coconut oil

Ingredients:

- ✓ 2 medium carrots, peeled and thinly sliced
- ✓ 6 radishes, trimmed and thinly sliced
- ✓ 2 tablespoons apple cider vinegar treatment - Salt, to taste.b.
- ✓ 1/3 cup coconut flakes, toasted
- ✓ 1 avocado, peeled, pitted and chopped

Directions:

❖ In a large bowl, add the kale, garlic, coconut amino acid, freshly squeezed lemon juice and olive oil and toss to coat well. Using your hands, generously rub in the kale. Add the coconut oil and toss to coat well. Set aside for about fifteen minutes, kneading occasionally.

❖ In another bowl, mix together the carrots, radishes and vinegar and set aside for about fifteen minutes, stirring occasionally. Add the carrot mixture to the inside of the bowl with the cabbage mixture and toss to combine. Serve with a garnish of coconut shavings and avocado.

## 148) WARM CHICKPEA SALAD

| **Preparation Time**: 10 minutes | **Cooking Time:** 10 minutes | **Servings: 4** |
|---|---|---|

Ingredients:

- ✓ 5 tablespoons virgin olive oil
- ✓ 1 large red onion, finely chopped
- ✓ 2 cloves garlic, minced
- ✓ 2 cans of chickpeas (15 oz.), rinsed and drained
- ✓ Pinch of red pepper flakes, crushed
- ✓ ½ teaspoon ground ginger

Ingredients:

- ✓ 1 tablespoon freshly squeezed lemon juice - Salt and freshly ground black pepper, to taste
- ✓ ¼ teaspoon paprika
- ✓ ½ teaspoon ground cumin
- ✓ 2 tablespoons fresh cilantro, chopped

Directions:

❖ In a skillet, heat 1 tablespoon oil over medium-low heat. Add the onion and garlic and sauté for about 5-7 minutes. Add the chickpeas, red pepper flakes and ground ginger and cook for about 1 minute. Add the fresh lemon juice and cook for about 1-2 minutes or until any liquid is absorbed.

❖ Transfer the chickpea mixture to the serving bowl. Add the remaining oil, paprika and cumin and gently, stir to combine. Serve warm with the cilantro garnish.

## 149) LENTIL AND BEET SALAD

| **Preparation Time**: 15 minutes | **Cooking Time:** about 20 minues | **Servings: 2-3** |
|---|---|---|

Ingredients:

For the salad:
- ✓ 2¾ cups water
- ✓ 1 cup puy lentils, rinsed - Salt, to taste
- ✓ 3 cooked beets, peeled and diced
- ✓ 2 shallots, chopped
- ✓ 2 tablespoons fresh parsley, chopped
- ✓ 2 tablespoons fresh mint leaves, chopped
- ✓ 2 tablespoons hazelnuts, chopped

Ingredients:

For the dressing:
- ✓ 1 (¾-inch) piece fresh ginger, chopped
- ✓ 1 teaspoon Dijon mustard
- ✓ 1/3 cup extra virgin olive oil essential
- ✓ 1 tablespoon apple cider vinegar - Salt and freshly ground black pepper, to taste

Directions:

❖ In a large skillet, add the water, lentils and salt over high heat and bring to a boil. Reduce heat to low and simmer for about 15-20 minutes or until all liquid is absorbed. Transfer the lentils right into a large bowl and set aside to cool.

❖ Add the remaining salad ingredients and toss to combine. In another bowl, add all dressing ingredients and beat until well combined. Place dressing on top of lentil mixture and stir until well combined. Serve immediately.

| 150) | CHICKEN SALAD WITH WALNUTS | |
|---|---|---|
| **Preparation Time**: 20 minutes | **Cooking Time**: | **Servings**: 6-8 |

| Ingredients: | Ingredients: |
|---|---|
| For the dressing:<br>✓ 2-3 tablespoons plain Greek yogurt<br>✓ 3 tablespoons Dijon mustard<br>✓ 2 tablespoons sunflower seeds<br>✓ 1 teaspoon turmeric powder<br>✓ ½-1 teaspoon turmeric powder<br>✓ ¼ teaspoon garlic powder<br>✓ ¼ teaspoon onion powder | ✓ Salt and freshly ground black pepper, to taste<br>For the salad:<br>✓ 4 cooked chicken breasts, shredded<br>✓ 2-3 celery stalks, chopped<br>✓ 7-10 sprigs fresh parsley<br>✓ 2 tablespoons dried cherries<br>✓ 2 tablespoons pecans<br>✓ 2 tablespoons slivered almonds |
| Directions:<br><br>❖ •For the dressing inside a bowl, add all the dressing ingredients and mix until well combined. In another large bowl, mix together salad ingredients. | ❖ Pour dressing over salad and toss to coat well. Serve immediately |

| 151) | THE CRAZY SALAD OF THE SOUTH | |
|---|---|---|
| **Preparation Time**: 10 minutes | **Cooking Time**: Nil | **Servings**: 2 |

| Ingredients: | Ingredients: |
|---|---|
| ✓ 5 cups romaine lettuce<br>✓ ½ cup sprouted black beans<br>✓ 1 cup cherry tomatoes, halved<br>✓ 1 avocado, diced | ✓ ¼ cup almonds, chopped<br>✓ ½ cup fresh cilantro<br>✓ ½ cup Salsa Fresca |
| Directions:<br><br>❖ Take a large bowl and add lettuce, tomatoes, beans, almonds, cilantro, avocado, Salsa Fresco Mix everything well and toss Divide salad into serving bowls and serve! Enjoy! | |

| 152) | CRISPY CABBAGE | |
|---|---|---|
| **Preparation Time**: 10 minutes | **Cooking Time**: 25 minutes | **Servings**: 4 |

| Ingredients: | Ingredients: |
|---|---|
| ✓ 3 cups kale, shredded and thoroughly washed, torn into 2-inch pieces<br>✓ 1 tablespoon extra-virgin olive oil | ✓ ½ teaspoon chili powder<br>✓ ¼ teaspoon sea salt |
| Directions:<br><br>❖ Prepare oven by preheating it to 300 degrees F. Line 2 baking sheets with baking paper and set aside. Pat the kale dry and transfer to a large bowl. | ❖ Add the olive oil and toss, making sure to cover the leaves well. Season the cabbage with salt, chili powder and toss. Divide cabbage between baking sheets and spread into a single layer. Bake for 25 minutes until crispy. Allow to cool for 5 minutes and serve. Enjoy! |

| 153) | CRAZY CARAMELIZED ONION | |
|---|---|---|
| **Preparation Time**: 10 minutes | **Cooking Time**: 9-10 hours | **Servings**: 4 |

Ingredients:

- ✓ 6 sliced onions
- ✓ 2 tablespoons oil

Ingredients:

- ✓ ½ teaspoon salt

Directions:

- ❖ Add the onions, oil and salt to your Slow Cooker. Close the lid and cook on LOW for 8 hours.

- ❖ Open the lid and continue to simmer for 1-2 hours until excess water has evaporated. Serve and enjoy!

| 154) | BROCCOLI CRUNCHIES | |
|---|---|---|
| **Preparation Time**: 10 minutes | **Cooking Time**: 3 hours | **Servings**: 4 |

Ingredients:

- ✓ 2 cups broccoli florets
- ✓ 2 ounces cream of celery
- ✓ 2 tablespoons cheddar cheese, shredded

Ingredients:

- ✓ 1 small yellow onion, chopped
- ✓ ¼ teaspoon Worcestershire sauce Salt and pepper to taste
- ✓ ½ tablespoon butter

Directions:

- ❖ Add the broccoli, cream cheese, onion and cheddar to the slow stove. Stir and season with salt and pepper.

- ❖ Put the lid on and cook on LOW for 3 hours. Serve and enjoy!

| 155) | A MIXTURE OF GREEN BEANS | |
|---|---|---|
| **Preparation Time**: 10 minutes | **Cooking Time**: 2 hours | **Servings**: 2 |

Ingredients:

- ✓ 4 cups green beans, cut
- ✓ 2 tablespoons butter, melted

Ingredients:

- ✓ 1 tablespoon date paste Salt and pepper to taste
- ✓ ¼ teaspoon coconut aminos

Directions:

- ❖ Add the green beans, date paste, pepper, salt, and coconut aminos to the slow stove; stir gently. Stir and put the lid on. Cook on LOW for 2 hours. Serve and enjoy!

| 156) | MIXED THREE MUSHROOMS | |
|---|---|---|
| **Preparation Time**: 15 minutes | **Cooking Time:** 17 minutes | **Servings: 3** |

Ingredients:

- ✓ 3 tablespoons extra virgin olive oil
- ✓ 3 portabella mushrooms, sliced
- ✓ 6 ounces shiitake mushrooms, sliced
- ✓ 7 1/2 ounces baby beech mushrooms
- ✓ 1 tablespoon fresh ginger, minced

Ingredients:

- ✓ 5 cloves garlic, minced
- ✓ 1 dried red pepper, crushed
- ✓ 2 teaspoons coconut aminos
- ✓ 1 teaspoon sesame oil

Directions:

- ❖ In a skillet, heat 1 tablespoon essential olive oil over medium heat.
- ❖ Add portabella mushrooms and cook, stirring occasionally, for about 4-5 minutes.
- ❖ Transfer mushrooms to a large bowl.
- ❖ In a similar skillet, heat 1 tablespoon of extra virgin olive oil over medium heat.
- ❖ Add the shiitake mushrooms and cook for about 4-5 minutes.
- ❖ Transfer the mushrooms to the large bowl with the portabella mushrooms.
- ❖ In a similar skillet, heat ½ tablespoon organic olive oil over medium heat.

- ❖ Add the porcini mushrooms and cook about 3-4 minutes.
- ❖ Transfer the mushrooms to the large bowl with portabella mushrooms.
- ❖ In the exact same pan, heat the remaining extra virgin olive oil over medium heat.
- ❖ Add the ginger, garlic and chili and sauté for about 1 minute.
- ❖ Add the mushroom mixture, coconut amino acid and sesame oil and stir until well combined.
- ❖ Cook for about 1 to 2 minutes.
- ❖ Serve hot.

| 157) | MIXED VEGETABLE STEW | |
|---|---|---|
| **Preparation Time**: 20 minutes | **Cooking Time:** 52 minutes | **Servings: 4** |

Ingredients:

- ✓ 2 tablespoons organic olive oil
- ✓ 1¼ cups yellow onion, chopped
- ✓ 1 tablespoon garlic, chopped
- ✓ 1 tablespoon chili paste
- ✓ 1½ tablespoons fresh turmeric, grated
- ✓ 1½ teaspoons ground cumin
- ✓ 1 teaspoon ground cinnamon

Ingredients:

- ✓ 1 cup carrots, peeled and coarsely chopped
- ✓ 1 cup cauliflower, coarsely chopped
- ✓ 2 cups broccoli, coarsely chopped
- ✓ 4 cups collard greens, coarsely chopped
- ✓ 1 cup coconut water
- ✓ 2 cups canned crushed tomatoes
- ✓ ¾ cup frozen peas, thawed - Salt and freshly ground black pepper, to taste

Directions:

- ❖ In a large skillet, heat the poi over medium heat.
- ❖ Add the onion and garlic and sauté about 10 minutes.
- ❖ Add the chili paste, turmeric, cumin and cinnamon and sauté for about 1 minute.
- ❖ Add the carrots and cook for about 3-4 minutes.
- ❖ Add the cauliflower and broccoli and cook for about 2-3 minutes.

- ❖ Add the kale while reducing the heat to low.
- ❖ Simmer for about 4 minutes.
- ❖ Add the coconut water and tomatoes and simmer over medium-high heat. Reduce heat to low and simmer, covered, for about thirty minutes. Add the peas, salt and black pepper and remove from heat. 11. Serve hot.

| **158)** | **STUFFED ZUCCHINIS** |
|---|---|

| **Preparation Time**: 20 minutes | **Cooking Time**: 30 minutes | **Servings**: 6 |
|---|---|---|

Ingredients:

- ✓ 6 medium zucchini, halved lengthwise
- ✓ Salt, to taste - 1½ baked potatoes, peeled and diced
- ✓ 4 teaspoons olive oil
- ✓ 2½ cups onion, chopped
- ✓ 1 Serrano pepper, chopped
- ✓ 2 cloves garlic, chopped
- ✓ 1½ tbsp. fresh ginger, chopped

Ingredients:

- ✓ 2 tablespoons chickpea flour
- ✓ 1 teaspoon ground cilantro
- ✓ ¼ teaspoon ground cumin
- ✓ ¼ teaspoon ground turmeric - fresh ground black pepper, to taste
- ✓ 1½ cups frozen green peas, thawed
- ✓ 2 tablespoons fresh cilantro, chopped

Directions:

- ❖ Preheat the oven to 375 degrees F
- ❖ Using a scoop, scoop out the flesh from the zucchini halves, leaving a shell about ¼ inch thick.
- ❖ In a shallow baking dish, arrange the zucchini halves, cut side up. Sprinkle the zucchini halves with a little salt. In a pot of boiling water, cook the potatoes for about 2 minutes

- ❖ Drain well and set aside. In a nonstick skillet, heat the oil over medium-high heat. Add the onion, Serrano, garlic and ginger and sauté for about 3 minutes. Reduce the heat to medium-low. Add the chickpea flour and spices and cook for about 5 minutes.
- ❖ Add the cooked potato, green peas and cilantro and remove from heat. Using a paper towel, pat the zucchini halves dry. Stuff the zucchini halves evenly with all the vegetable mixture, Bake, covered for about 20 minutes.

| **159)** | **VEGETABLES WITH CHICKPEAS** |
|---|---|

| **Preparation Time**: 20 minutes | **Cooking Time**: 25 minutes | **Servings**: 2 |
|---|---|---|

Ingredients:

- ✓ ¼ cup onion, chopped
- ✓ 1 piece fresh ginger (1 inch), chopped
- ✓ 4 cloves garlic, minced
- ✓ 2-3 tablespoons water
- ✓ 1 teaspoon organic olive oil
- ✓ ½ teaspoon ground coriander
- ✓ ½ teaspoon ground cumin
- ✓ ½ teaspoon ground turmeric
- ✓ ¼ teaspoon ground cardamom
- ✓ ¼ teaspoon ground cinnamon
- ✓ 1/3 teaspoon ground red cayenne pepper

Ingredients:

- ✓ ½ cup coconut milk
- ✓ 3 tablespoons almond butter
- ✓ ¾ cup vegetable broth
- ✓ 1 (15-ounce) can chickpeas, rinsed and drained
- ✓ ½ cup zucchini, sliced
- ✓ ½ cup carrots, peeled and sliced
- ✓ ½ cup red bell bell pepper, seedless and sliced - Crushed red pepper flakes, to taste - Salt and freshly ground black pepper, to taste
- ✓ 1 teaspoon fresh lime juice
- ✓ ¼ cup fresh cilantro, chopped

Directions:

- ❖ In blender, add onion, ginger, garlic and water and pulse until smooth. In a skillet, heat oil over medium heat. Add the spices and sauté for about 30 seconds. Reduce the temperature to medium-low. Add the onion mixture and sauté for about 7-9 minutes.
- ❖ Add the coconut milk and almond butter and stir to mix well. Increase the heat to medium-high.

- ❖ Add the broth, chickpeas, vegetables, red pepper flakes, salt and black pepper and bring to a boil for about 4 minutes.
- ❖ Reduce the heat to medium-low and simmer for about 5 minutes. Add the lime juice and cilantro and simmer for about 3-4 minutes.

| 160) | THREE BEAN SPICY CHILI | |
|---|---|---|
| **Preparation Time**: 15 minutes | **Cooking Time**: 60 minutes | **Servings: 6** |

**Ingredients:**

- ✓ 1 teaspoon dried oregano, crushed
- ✓ 1 tablespoon red chili powder
- ✓ 1 tablespoon red pepper flakes, crushed
- ✓ 2 teaspoons ground cumin
- ✓ 1 teaspoon ground turmeric
- ✓ 1 teaspoon onion powder
- ✓ 1 teaspoon garlic powder
- ✓ 1 teaspoon paprika - Salt and freshly ground black pepper, to taste-
- ✓ 2 tablespoons extra virgin olive oil
- ✓ 1 red bell bell pepper, seeded and chopped

**Ingredients:**

- ✓ 1 green bell bell pepper, seeded and chopped
- ✓ 3 large celery stalks, chopped
- ✓ 1 shallot, chopped
- ✓ 3 cloves garlic, chopped
- ✓ 1 (28-ounce) can unsalted diced tomatoes
- ✓ 4 cups water
- ✓ 1 (16-ounce) can kidney beans, rinsed and drained
- ✓ 1 (16-ounce) can cannellini beans, rinsed and drained
- ✓ 1 (8-ounce) can black beans, rinsed and drained –
- ✓ 1 jalapeño bell pepper, seeded and chopped

**Directions:**

- ❖ For the spice mixture in a bowl, mix all ingredients together. Keep aside.
- ❖ In a large skillet, heat oil over medium heat. Add peppers, celery, shallots and garlic and sauté about 8-10 minutes.

- ❖ Add the spice mixture, tomatoes and water and bring to a boil. Simmer for about 20 minutes. Add the beans and jalapeño pepper and simmer for about 30 minutes. Serve hot.

| 161) | ROASTED ONIONS AND GREEN BEANS | |
|---|---|---|
| **Preparation Time**: 10 minutes | **Cooking Time**: 15 minutes | **Servings: 6** |

**Ingredients:**

- ✓ 1 yellow onion, cut into rings
- ✓ ½ teaspoon onion powder

**Ingredients:**

- ✓ 2 tablespoons coconut flour
- ✓ 1 1/3 pounds fresh green beans, cut and chopped

**Directions:**

- ❖ Take a large bowl and mix the sunflower seeds with the onion powder and coconut flour. Add the onion rings. Mix well to coat. Spread the rings in the baking dish, lined with baking paper.

- ❖ Drizzle with a little oil. Bake for 10 minutes at 400 degrees F. Parboil the green beans for 3 to 5 minutes in boiling water. Drain and serve the beans with the baked onion rings. Serve hot and enjoy!

| 162) | CAULIFLOWER RICE | |
|---|---|---|
| **Preparation Time**: 5 minutes | **Cooking Time**: 6 minutes | **Servings**: 2 |

Ingredients:

- ✓ 1 head of grated cauliflower
- ✓ 1 tablespoon of coconut aminos
- ✓ 1 pinch of sunflower seeds

Ingredients:

- ✓ 1 pinch of black pepper
- ✓ 1 tablespoon of garlic powder
- ✓ 1 tablespoon of sesame oil

Directions:

- ❖ Add the cauliflower to a food processor and grate it. Take a frying pan and add the sesame oil, let it heat over medium heat.

- ❖ Add the grated cauliflower and pour in the coconut aminos. Cook for 4-6 minutes. Season and enjoy!

| 163) | AMAZING CREAMY GREEN CABBAGE | |
|---|---|---|
| **Preparation Time**: 10 minutes | **Cooking Time**: 10 minutes | **Servings**: 4 |

Ingredients:

- ✓ 2 ounces almond butter
- ✓ 1 ½ pounds kale, shredded

Ingredients:

- ✓ 1 ¼ cups coconut cream Sunflower seeds and pepper to taste
- ✓ 8 tablespoons fresh parsley, chopped

Directions:

- ❖ Take a skillet and put it over medium heat, add the almond butter and let it melt. Add the kale and sauté it until it turns brown. Add the cream and turn the heat down to low.

- ❖ Allow to simmer. Season with sunflower seeds and pepper. Garnish with parsley and serve. Enjoy!

| 164) | ROAST GREEN BEANS | |
|---|---|---|
| **Preparation Time**: 10 minutes | **Cooking Time**: 20 minutes | **Servings**: 4 |

Ingredients:

- ✓ 1 whole egg
- ✓ 2 tablespoons olive oil Sunflower seeds and pepper to taste

Ingredients:

- ✓ 1 pound fresh green beans
- ✓ 5 ½ tablespoons grated Parmesan cheese

Directions:

- ❖ Preheat oven to 400 degrees F. Take a bowl and beat eggs with oil and spices. Add the beans and mix well. Stir in the Parmesan cheese and pour the mixture into the baking dish (lined with baking paper).

- ❖ Bake for 15-20 minutes. Serve warm and enjoy!

## 165) TOMATO DISH

| **Preparation Time**: 10 minutes + cooling time | **Cooking Time**: Nil | **Servings**: 8 |
|---|---|---|

Ingredients:

- ✓ 1/3 cup olive oil
- ✓ 1 teaspoon sunflower seeds
- ✓ 2 tablespoons onion, chopped
- ✓ ¼ teaspoon pepper
- ✓ ½ garlic, chopped

Ingredients:

- ✓ 1 tablespoon fresh parsley, chopped
- ✓ 3 large fresh tomatoes, sliced
- ✓ 1 teaspoon dried basil
- ✓ ¼ cup red wine vinegar

Directions:

- ❖ Take a shallow dish and arrange the tomatoes on it. Add the rest of the ingredients to a glass jar, cover the jar and shake it well.

- ❖ Pour the mixture over the tomato slices. Allow to cool for 2-3 hours. Serve.

## 166) FRESH CHICKPEAS AND SPINACH BEANS

| **Preparation Time**: 5-10 minutes | **Cooking Time**: Nil | **Servings**: 4 |
|---|---|---|

Ingredients:

- ✓ 1 tablespoon olive oil
- ✓ ½ onion, diced
- ✓ 10 ounces spinach, chopped

Ingredients:

- ✓ 12 ounces chickpeas
- ✓ ½ teaspoon cumin

Directions:

- ❖ Take a skillet and add the olive oil, let it heat over medium-low heat. Add the onions, chickpeas and cook for 5 minutes. Add the spinach, cumin, chickpeas and season with the sunflower seeds.

- ❖ Use a spoon to gently mash. Cook thoroughly until heated through, enjoy!

## 167) CELERIAC PUREE

| **Preparation Time**: 10 minutes | **Cooking Time**: 20 minutes | **Servings**: 4 |
|---|---|---|

Ingredients:

- ✓ 2 washed, peeled and diced celeriac
- ✓ 2 teaspoons extra virgin olive oil

Ingredients:

- ✓ 1 tablespoon honey
- ✓ ½ teaspoon nutmeg powder Sunflower seeds and pepper to taste

Directions:

- ❖ Preheat oven to 400 degrees F. Line a baking sheet with aluminum foil and set aside. Take a large bowl and mix the celeriac with the olive oil. Spread the celeriac evenly on a baking sheet. Roast for 20 minutes until tender.

- ❖ Transfer to a large bowl. Add the honey and nutmeg. Use a potato masher to mash the mixture until fluffy. Season with sunflower seeds and pepper. Serve and enjoy!

## 168) MEDITERRANEAN DISH OF KALE

| **Preparation Time**: 15 minutes | **Cooking Time:** 10 minutes | **Servings: 6** |
|---|---|---|

Ingredients:

- ✓ 12 cups cabbage, chopped
- ✓ 2 tablespoons lemon juice

Ingredients:

- ✓ 1 tablespoon olive oil
- ✓ 1 teaspoon coconut aminos Sunflower seeds and pepper as needed

Directions:

- ❖ Add a steamer insert to the pot. Fill the pot with water to the bottom of the steamer. Cover and bring the water to a boil (medium-high heat). Add the cabbage to the insert and steam for 7-8 minutes.

- ❖ Take a large bowl and add the lemon juice, olive oil, sunflower seeds, coconut amino acid and pepper. Mix well and add the steamed cabbage to the bowl. Stir and serve.

## 169) PORTOBELLO MUSHROOMS SEEMINGLY EASY

| **Preparation Time**: 10 minutes | **Cooking Time:** 10 minutes | **Servings: 4** |
|---|---|---|

Ingredients:

- ✓ 12 cherry tomatoes
- ✓ 2 ounces shallots

Ingredients:

- ✓ 4 portabella mushrooms
- ✓ 4 ounces almond butter Sunflower seeds and pepper to taste

Directions:

- ❖ Take a large skillet and melt the almond butter over medium heat. Add the mushrooms and sauté for 3 minutes.

- ❖ Add the cherry tomatoes and shallots. Sauté for 5 minutes. Season accordingly. Sauté until the vegetables are tender. Enjoy!

## 170) CLASSIC GUACAMOLE

| **Preparation Time**: 15 minutes | **Cooking Time:** Nil | **Servings: 6** |
|---|---|---|

Ingredients:

- ✓ 3 large, ripe avocados
- ✓ 1 large red onion, peeled and diced
- ✓ 4 tablespoons freshly squeezed lime juice

Ingredients:

- ✓ Sunflower seeds as needed
- ✓ Freshly ground black pepper as needed
- ✓ Cayenne pepper as needed

Directions:

- ❖ Halve the avocados and discard the pit. Scoop out the flesh from 3 avocado halves and transfer to a large bowl. Mash with a fork. Add 2 tablespoons lime juice and toss to combine.

- ❖ Dice the remaining avocado flesh (the remaining half) and transfer to another bowl. Add the remaining juice and toss to combine. Add the diced pulp to the mashed pulp and stir. Add chopped onions and toss to combine. Season with sunflower seeds, pepper and cayenne pepper. Serve and enjoy!

| 171) | ELEGANT CASHEW SAUCE | |
|---|---|---|
| **Preparation Time**: 5 minutes | **Cooking Time**: Nil | **Servings**: 4 |

Ingredients:

- ✓ 3 ounces cashews
- ✓ ¼ cup water
- ✓ ½ cup olive oil
- ✓ 1 tablespoon lemon juice

Ingredients:

- ✓ ½ teaspoon onion powder
- ✓ ½ teaspoon sunflower seeds
- ✓ 1 pinch cayenne pepper

Directions:

❖ Add the walnuts to the blender and process. Add the remaining ingredients (except the oil) and process until smooth.

❖ Add a little oil and blend. Serve as needed!

| 172) | BUTTERY GREEN CABBAGE WITH ALMONDS | |
|---|---|---|
| **Preparation Time**: 10 minutes | **Cooking Time**: 15 minutes | **Servings**: 4 |

Ingredients:

- ✓ 1 1/2 pounds shredded green cabbage
- ✓ 3 ounces almond butter Sunflower seeds and pepper to taste

Ingredients:

- ✓ 1 tablespoon whipped cream

Directions:

❖ Take a large skillet and place it over medium heat. Add the almond butter and melt it.

❖ Add the kale and sauté for 15 minutes. Season accordingly. Serve with a spoonful of cream. Enjoy!

| 173) | BRUSSELS FEVER | |
|---|---|---|
| **Preparation Time**: 10 minutes | **Cooking Time**: 20 minutes | **Servings**: 4 |

Ingredients:

- ✓ 2 tablespoons olive oil
- ✓ 1 yellow onion, chopped
- ✓ 2 pounds Brussels sprouts, cut and halved

Ingredients:

- ✓ 4 cups vegetable stock
- ✓ ¼ cup coconut cream

Directions:

❖ Take a saucepan and place it over medium heat. Add the oil and let it heat up. Add the onion and stir for 3 minutes. Add the Brussels sprouts and stir, cook for 2 minutes.

❖ Add the broth and black pepper, stir and bring to a boil. Cook for an additional 20 minutes. Use an immersion blender to make the soup creamy. Add the coconut cream and mix well. Pour into soup bowls and serve. Enjoy!

| 174) | JAY WITH MANGO CHUTNEY | |
|---|---|---|
| **Preparation Time**: 10 minutes | **Cooking Time:** 3 hours 10 minutes | **Servings: 4** |

Ingredients:

- ✓ 1 large acorn squash
- ✓ ¼ cup mango chutney

Ingredients:

- ✓ ¼ cup flaked coconut Salt and pepper to taste

Directions:

- ❖ Cut squash into quarters and remove seeds, discard pulp. Spray the pot with olive oil. Transfer the squash to the Slow Cooker pot and put the lid on.

- ❖ Take a bowl and add the coconut and chutney, mix well and divide the mixture in the center of the squash. Season well. Put the lid on and cook on LOW for 2-3 hours. Enjoy!

| 175) | PURE MAPLE GLAZED CARROTS | |
|---|---|---|
| **Preparation Time**: 10 minutes | **Cooking Time:** 8 hours | **Servings: 6** |

Ingredients:

- ✓ ¼ cup pure maple syrup
- ✓ ½ teaspoon ground ginger
- ✓ ¼ teaspoon ground nutmeg

Ingredients:

- ✓ ½ teaspoon salt Juice of 1 orange
- ✓ 1 pound baby carrots

Directions:

- ❖ Take a small bowl and whisk the syrup, nutmeg, ginger, salt and orange juice. Add the carrots to your Slow Cooker and pour in the maple syrup. Stir to coat.

- ❖ Close the lid and cook on LOW for 8 hours. Serve and enjoy!

| 176) | PINEAPPLE RICE | |
|---|---|---|
| **Preparation Time**: 10 minutes | **Cooking Time:** 2 hours | **Servings: 2** |

Ingredients:

- ✓ 1 cup rice
- ✓ 2 cups water
- ✓ 1 small cauliflower, florets separated and chopped

Ingredients:

- ✓ ½ small pineapple, peeled and chopped Salt and pepper to taste
- ✓ 1 teaspoon olive oil

Directions:

- ❖ Add the rice, cauliflower, pineapple, water, oil, salt and pepper to your Slow Cooker. Stir gently.

- ❖ Put the lid on and cook on HIGH for 2 hours. Mash the rice with a fork and season with more salt and pepper if needed. Divide among serving plates and enjoy!

## 177) NEW POTATOES

| **Preparation Time**: 10 minutes | **Cooking Time**: 35 minutes | **Servings**: 4 |
|---|---|---|

Ingredients:

- ✓ 2 pounds new yellow potatoes, peeled and cut into wedges
- ✓ 2 tablespoons extra virgin olive oil
- ✓ 2 teaspoons fresh rosemary, chopped

Ingredients:

- ✓ 1 teaspoon garlic powder
- ✓ ½ teaspoon freshly ground black pepper and sunflower seeds

Directions:

- ❖ Preheat the oven to 400 degrees F. Line a baking sheet with aluminum foil and set aside. Take a large bowl and add the potatoes, olive oil, garlic, rosemary, sea sunflower seeds and pepper.

- ❖ Spread the potatoes in a single layer on a baking sheet and bake for 35 minutes. Serve and enjoy

## 178) TENDER RICE WITH COCONUT AND CAULIFLOWER WITH CHILLI

| **Preparation Time**: 20 minutes | **Cooking Time**: 20 minutes | **Servings**: 4 |
|---|---|---|

Ingredients:

- ✓ 3 cups cauliflower, shredded
- ✓ 2/3 cup whole almond coconut milk

Ingredients:

- ✓ 1-2 teaspoons sriracha paste
- ✓ ¼- ½ teaspoon onion powder Sunflower seeds as needed Fresh basil for garnish

Directions:

- ❖ Take a skillet and place it over medium low heat. Add all the ingredients and stir until they are completely combined. Cook for about 5-10 minutes, making sure you have the lid on.

- ❖ Remove the lid and continue cooking until the excess liquid is absorbed. Once the rice is soft and creamy, enjoy!

## 179) THE EXQUISITE SPAGHETTI

| **Preparation Time**: 5 minutes | **Cooking Time**: 7-8 hours | **Servings**: 6 |
|---|---|---|

Ingredients:

- ✓ 1 spaghetti squash

Ingredients:

- ✓ 2 cups water

Directions:

- ❖ Wash the pumpkin thoroughly with water and rinse it well. Poke 5-6 holes in the squash with a fork. Place the squash in the slow stove. Put the lid on and cook on LOW for 7-8 hours.

- ❖ Remove pumpkin to cutting board and let cool. Cut the squash in half and discard the seeds. Use two forks and scrape out the pumpkin strands and transfer to a bowl. Serve and enjoy!

## 180) EASY CAULIFLOWER PEPPER JACK

| **Preparation Time**: 10 minutes | **Cooking Time**: 3 hours 35 minutes | **Servings**: 6 |
|---|---|---|

| Ingredients: | Ingredients: |
|---|---|
| ✓ 1 head of cauliflower<br>✓ ¼ cup whipping cream<br>✓ 4 ounces cream cheese<br>✓ ½ teaspoon pepper | ✓ 1 teaspoon salt<br>✓ 2 tablespoons butter<br>✓ 4 ounces pepper jack cheese |
| ❖ Grease slow stove and add ingredients listed. Stir and place lid on, cook on LOW for 3 hours. | ❖ Remove lid and add cheese, stir. Put the lid back on and cook for 1 more hour. Enjoy. |

## 181) SIMPLE RICE RISOTTO WITH MUSHROOMS

| **Preparation Time**: 5 minutes | **Cooking Time**: 15 minutes | **Servings**: 4 |
|---|---|---|

| Ingredients: | Ingredients: |
|---|---|
| ✓ 4 1/2 cups cauliflower, mashed<br>✓ 3 tablespoons coconut oil<br>✓ 1 pound Portobello mushrooms, thinly sliced<br>✓ 1 pound white mushrooms, thinly sliced<br>✓ 2 shallots, diced | ✓ ¼ cup organic vegetable broth Sunflower seeds and pepper to taste<br>✓ 3 tablespoons chives, chopped<br>✓ 4 tablespoons almond butter<br>✓ ½ cup kite/cashew cottage cheese, grated |
| ❖ Use a food processor and pulse the cauliflower florets until they are reduced to a mush. Take a large saucepan and heat 2 tablespoons of oil over medium-high heat.<br>❖ Add the mushrooms and sauté for 3 minutes until the mushrooms are tender. Clear the casserole of the mushrooms and liquid and set aside. Add the remaining 1 tablespoon of oil to the skillet. Cough up the scallions and cook for 60 seconds. | ❖ Add the rice to the cauliflower, stir for 2 minutes until coated with oil. Add the broth to the embroidered cauliflower and stir for 5 minutes. Remove the pot from the heat and stir in the mushrooms and liquid.<br>❖ Add the chives, almond butter and parmesan cheese. Season with sunflower seeds and pepper. Serve and enjoy! |

## 182) ALMOND AND BEANS IN BUBBLE

| **Preparation Time**: 10 minutes | **Cooking Time**: 20 minutes | **Servings**: 4 |
|---|---|---|

| Ingredients: | Ingredients: |
|---|---|
| ✓ 1 pound fresh green beans, ends cut off<br>✓ 1 ½ tablespoons olive oil<br>✓ ¼ tablespoon sunflower seeds | ✓ 1 ½ tablespoons fresh dill, chopped Juice of 1 lemon<br>✓ ¼ cup chopped almonds Sunflower seeds as needed |

| Directions: | |
|---|---|
| ❖ Preheat the oven to 400 degrees F. Add the green beans with the olive oil and also the sunflower seeds. Then spread them in a single layer on a large baking sheet. | ❖ Roast for 10 minutes and stir, then roast for another 8-10 minutes. Remove from the oven and continue to toss with the lemon juice along with the dill.<br>❖ Top with crushed almonds and some slivered sunflower seeds and serve. |

## 183)   LEMON SPROUTS

| **Preparation Time**: 10 minutes | **Cooking Time**: no | **Servings**: 4 |
|---|---|---|

| Ingredients: | Ingredients: |
|---|---|
| ✓ 1 pound Brussels sprouts, chopped and shredded<br>✓ 8 tablespoons olive oil | ✓ 1 lemon, juice and zest Sunflower seeds and pepper to taste<br>✓ ¾ cup seed mix and spicy almonds |
| ❖ Take a bowl and mix in the lemon juice, sunflower seeds, pepper and olive oil. Mix well. | ❖ Add the shredded Brussels sprouts and toss to combine. Let stand for 10 minutes. Add the walnuts and stir. Serve and enjoy! |

## 184)   DELICIOUS GARLIC TOMATOES

| **Preparation Time**: 10 minutes | **Cooking Time**: 50 minutes | **Servings**: 4 |
|---|---|---|

| Ingredients: | Ingredients: |
|---|---|
| ✓ 4 garlic cloves, crushed<br>✓ 1 pound mixed cherry tomatoes | ✓ 3 sprigs thyme, chopped Pinch of sunflower seeds Black pepper to taste<br>✓ ¼ cup olive oil |
| ❖ Preheat the oven to 325 degrees F. Take a baking sheet and add the tomatoes, olive oil and thyme. | ❖ Season with sunflower seeds and pepper and toss to combine. Bake for 50 minutes. Divide the tomatoes and cooking juices and serve. Enjoy! |

## 185)   SPICY WASABI MAYONNAISE

| **Preparation Time**: 15 minutes | **Cooking Time**: no | **Servings**: 4 |
|---|---|---|

| | |
|---|---|
| ✓ 1 cup mayonnaise | ✓ ½ tablespoon wasabi paste |
| ❖ Take a bowl and mix the wasabi paste and mayonnaise together. Mix well. Allow to cool and use as needed | |

## 186)   SPICY CABBAGE CHIPS

| **Preparation Time**: 10 minutes | **Cooking Time**: 25 minutes | **Servings**: 4 |
|---|---|---|

| Ingredients: | Ingredients: |
|---|---|
| ✓ 3 cups kale, shredded and thoroughly washed, torn into 2-inch pieces<br>✓ 1 tablespoon extra-virgin olive oil | ✓ ½ teaspoon chili powder<br>✓ ¼ teaspoon sea sunflower seeds |
| ❖ Preheat oven to 300 degrees F. Line 2 baking sheets with baking paper and set aside. Dry the kale completely and transfer to a large bowl.<br>❖ Add the olive oil and toss to combine. Make sure each leaf is covered. Season the cabbage with chili powder and sunflower seeds, toss again. | ❖ Divide cabbage between baking sheets and spread into a single layer. Bake for 25 minutes until crispy. Cool the chips for 5 minutes and serve. Enjoy! |

| 187) | THE CHICKPEA EXTRAVAGANZA | |
|---|---|---|
| **Preparation Time**: 10 minutes | **Cooking Time**: Nil | **Servings: 5** |

| Ingredients: | Ingredients: |
|---|---|
| ✓ 1 can of chickpeas<br>✓ 1 tablespoon olive oil<br>✓ 1 teaspoon sunflower seeds | ✓ 1 teaspoon garlic powder<br>✓ ½ teaspoon paprika |

| Directions: | ❖ Stir in olive oil, sunflower seeds, garlic powder, paprika and mix well. Spread on a baking sheet. Bake for 20 minutes. Turn chickpeas so they are well roasted. |
|---|---|
| ❖ Preheat oven to 375 degrees F. Line a baking sheet with a silicone baking mat. Drain and rinse chickpeas, pat dry and place in a large bowl. | ❖ Return to oven and bake for another 25 minutes at 375 degrees F. Let cool and enjoy! |

| 188) | APPLE SLICES | |
|---|---|---|
| **Preparation Time**: 10 minutes | **Cooking Time**: 10 minutes | **Servings: 4** |

| Ingredients: | Ingredients: |
|---|---|
| ✓ 1 cup coconut oil<br>✓ ¼ cup date paste | ✓ 2 tablespoons ground cinnamon<br>✓ 4 granny smith apples, peeled and sliced, cored |

| Directions: | ❖ Stir the cinnamon and date paste into the oil. Add the chopped apples and cook for 5-8 minutes until crispy. Serve and enjoy! |
|---|---|
| ❖ Take a large skillet and place it over medium heat. Add the oil and let the oil heat up. | |

| 189) | A DELICIOUS JAPANESE CABBAGE DISH | |
|---|---|---|
| **Preparation Time**: 25 minutes | **Cooking Time**: Nil | **Servings: 6** |

| Ingredients: | Ingredients: |
|---|---|
| ✓ 3 tablespoons sesame oil<br>✓ 3 tablespoons rice vinegar<br>✓ 1 clove garlic, minced<br>✓ 1 teaspoon fresh ginger root, grated<br>✓ 1 teaspoon sunflower seeds | ✓ 1 teaspoon pepper<br>✓ ½ large head cabbage, shredded and chopped<br>✓ 1 bunch green onions, thinly sliced<br>✓ 1 cup almond slivers<br>✓ ¼ cup toasted sesame seeds |

| Directions: | ❖ Mix well to make sure the kale is coated well. Allow to cool and enjoy! |
|---|---|
| ❖ Add all of the listed ingredients to a large bowl, making sure to add the wet ingredients first, followed by the dry ingredients. | |

| 190) MESMERIZING BRUSSELS AND PISTACHIOS | | |
|---|---|---|
| **Preparation Time**: 15 minutes | **Cooking Time:** 15 minutes | **Servings: 4** |

| Ingredients: | Ingredients: |
|---|---|
| ✓ 1 pound Brussels sprouts, hard underside cut in half lengthwise<br>✓ 1 tablespoon extra virgin olive oil Sunflower seeds and pepper to taste | ✓ ½ cup toasted pistachios, chopped<br>✓ Juice of ½ lemon |
| Directions:<br><br>❖ Preheat oven to 400 degrees F. Line a baking sheet with aluminum foil and set aside. Take a large bowl and add Brussels sprouts with olive oil and coat well. | ❖ Season sea sunflower seeds, pepper, scatter vegetables evenly over foil. Bake for 15 minutes until lightly caramelized. Remove from oven and transfer to a serving bowl.<br>❖ Stir in pistachios and lemon juice. Serve warm and enjoy! |

| 191) GARLIC AND KALE DISH | | |
|---|---|---|
| **Preparation Time**: 5 minutes | **Cooking Time:** 10 minutes | **Servings: 4** |

| Ingredients: | Ingredients: |
|---|---|
| ✓ 1 bunch of cabbage<br>✓ 2 tablespoons olive oil | ✓ 4 cloves of garlic, minced |
| Directions:<br><br>❖ Carefully cut the cabbage into bite-sized portions, making sure to remove the stem. Discard the stems. | ❖ Take a large pot and place it over medium heat. Add the olive oil and let the oil heat up. Add the garlic and stir for 2 minutes. Add the kale and cook for 5-10 minutes. Serve. |

| 192) SATISFYING PORRIDGE OF HONEY AND COCONUT | | |
|---|---|---|
| **Preparation Time**: 10 minutes | **Cooking Time:** 8 hours | **Servings: 8** |

| Ingredients: | Ingredients: |
|---|---|
| ✓ 4 cups light coconut milk<br>✓ 3 cups apple juice<br>✓ 2 ¼ cups coconut flour | ✓ 1 teaspoon cinnamon powder<br>✓ ¼ cup honey |
| Directions:<br><br>❖ In a Slow Cooker, add the coconut milk, apple juice, flour, cinnamon and honey. | ❖ Mix well. Close the lid and cook on LOW for 8 hours. Open the lid and stir. Serve with an additional topping of fresh fruit. Enjoy! |

| 193) | GINGER AND ORANGE BEETS | |
|---|---|---|
| **Preparation Time**: 20 minutes | **Cooking Time:** 8 hours | **Servings: 6** |

Ingredients:

- ✓ 2 pounds beets, peeled and cut into wedges Juice of 2 oranges Zest of 1 orange
- ✓ 1 teaspoon fresh ginger, grated
- ✓ 1 tablespoon honey

Ingredients:

- ✓ 1 tablespoon apple cider vinegar
- ✓ 1/8 teaspoon fresh ground black pepper Sea salt

Directions:

- ❖ Add the beets, zest, orange juice, ginger, honey, pepper, salt and vinegar to your Slow Cooker.

- ❖ Stir well. Close the lid and cook on LOW for 8 hours. Serve and enjoy!

| 194) | CREATIVE DISH WITH LEMON AND BROCCOLI | |
|---|---|---|
| **Preparation Time**: 10 minutes | **Cooking Time:** 15 minutes | **Servings: 6** |

Ingredients:

- ✓ 2 heads of broccoli, separated into florets
- ✓ 2 teaspoons extra virgin olive oil
- ✓ 1 teaspoon sunflower seeds

Ingredients:

- ✓ ½ teaspoon black pepper
- ✓ 1 clove garlic, minced
- ✓ ½ teaspoon lemon juice

Directions:

- ❖ Preheat oven to 400 degrees F. Take a large bowl and add broccoli florets. Drizzle olive oil and season with pepper, sunflower seeds and garlic.

- ❖ Spread broccoli in a single even layer on a baking sheet. Bake for 15-20 minutes until fork tender. Squeeze lemon juice over top. Serve and enjoy!

| 195) | CAULIFLOWER CAKES | |
|---|---|---|
| **Preparation Time**: 10 minutes | **Cooking Time:** 10 minutes | **Servings: 4** |

Ingredients:

- ✓ 4 cups cauliflower, florets cut
- ✓ 1 cup ricotta kite/ cashew cheese, grated
- ✓ 2 eggs, lightly beaten
- ✓ 1 teaspoon paprika

Ingredients:

- ✓ 1 teaspoon chili powder Sunflower seeds and pepper to taste
- ✓ ½ cup fresh parsley, chopped
- ✓ 1 tablespoon olive oil

Directions:

- ❖ Add the cauliflower, cheese, paprika, eggs, chili, sunflower seeds, pepper and parsley to a large bowl.

- ❖ Mix well. Pour olive oil into a skillet and place over medium-high heat. Form the cauliflower mixture into 12 even patties.
- ❖ Once the oil is hot, fry the patties until both sides are golden brown. Serve hot and enjoy!

| 196) APPLE SLICES | | |
|---|---|---|
| **Preparation Time**: 10 minutes | **Cooking Time:** 10 minutes | **Servings: 4** |

| Ingredients: | Ingredients: |
|---|---|
| ✓  1 cup coconut oil<br>✓  ¼ cup date paste | ✓  2 tablespoons ground cinnamon<br>✓  4 Granny Smith apples, peeled and sliced, cored |
| **Directions:**<br><br>❖  Take a large skillet and place it over medium heat. Add the oil and let the oil heat up. | ❖  Stir the cinnamon and date paste into the oil. Add the sliced apples and cook for 5-8 minutes until crispy. Serve and enjoy! |

| 197) CRUNCHY GARLIC AND MUSHROOMS | | |
|---|---|---|
| **Preparation Time**: 10 minutes | **Cooking Time:** 8 hours | **Servings: 6** |

| Ingredients: | Ingredients: |
|---|---|
| ✓  ¼ cup vegetable stock<br>✓  2 tablespoons extra-virgin olive oil<br>✓  1 tablespoon Dijon mustard<br>✓  1 teaspoon dried thyme<br>✓  1 teaspoon sea salt | ✓  ½ teaspoon dried rosemary<br>✓  ¼ teaspoon freshly ground black pepper<br>✓  2 pounds cremini mushrooms, cleaned<br>✓  6 cloves garlic, chopped<br>✓  ¼ cup fresh parsley, chopped |
| **Directions:**<br><br>❖  Take a small bowl and whisk together the vegetable broth, mustard, olive oil, salt, thyme, pepper and rosemary. Add the mushrooms, garlic and broth mix to your Slow Cooker. | ❖  Close the lid and cook on LOW for 8 hours. Open the lid and stir in the parsley. Serve and enjoy! |

| 198) THE BRUSSELS PLATE | | |
|---|---|---|
| **Preparation Time**: 15 minutes | **Cooking Time:** 4 hours | **Servings: 4** |

| Ingredients: | Ingredients: |
|---|---|
| ✓  1 pound Brussels sprouts, bottom cut off<br>✓  1 tablespoon olive oil | ✓  1 ½ tablespoons Dijon mustard Salt and pepper to taste<br>✓  ½ teaspoon dried tarragon |
| **Directions:**<br><br>❖  Add the Brussels sprouts, mustard, water, salt and pepper to your Slow Cooker and add the dried tarragon. Stir well and cover. | ❖  Cook on LOW for 5 hours, making sure to continue cooking until the Brussels sprouts are tender. Stir well and arrange. Add the Dijon on top of the Brussels sprouts. Enjoy! |

## 199) CABBAGE AND CARROTS WITH TAHINI DRESSING

| Preparation Time: 15 minutes | Cooking Time: Nil | Servings: 1 |
| --- | --- | --- |

Ingredients:

- ✓ Handful of cabbage
- ✓ 1 tablespoon tahnini
- ✓ ½ head lettuce Pinch of garlic powder

Ingredients:

- ✓ 1 tablespoon olive oil Juice of ½ lime
- ✓ 1 carrot, grated

Directions:

- ❖ Add the cabbage and roughly chopped lettuce to a bowl. Add the grated carrots to the greens and mix.

- ❖ Take a small bowl and add the remaining ingredients, mix well. Pour the dressing over the greens and toss. Enjoy!

## 200) JUICY VEGETABLES FOR SUMMER

| Preparation Time: 10 minutes | Cooking Time: 3 hours 5 minutes | Servings: 6 |
| --- | --- | --- |

Ingredients:

- ✓ 1 cup grape tomatoes
- ✓ 2 cups okra
- ✓ 1 cup mushrooms
- ✓ 2 cups yellow peppers
- ✓ 1 ½ cups red onions

Ingredients:

- ✓ 2 ½ cups zucchini
- ✓ ½ cup olive oil
- ✓ ½ cup balsamic vinegar
- ✓ 1 tablespoon fresh thyme, chopped
- ✓ 2 tablespoons fresh basil, chopped

- ❖ Slice and chop okra, onions, tomatoes, zucchini, mushrooms. Add vegetables to a large container and mix. Take another dish and add oil and vinegar, stir in thyme and basil.

- ❖ Place vegetables in Slow Cooker and pour in marinade. Stir well. Close the lid and cook for 3 hours on HIGH, making sure to stir after every hour.

## 201) BEANS AND CILANTRO

| Preparation Time: 5 minutes | Cooking Time: Nil | Servings: 6 |
| --- | --- | --- |

Ingredients:

- ✓ 1 can beans, drained and rinsed
- ✓ ½ English cucumber, chopped
- ✓ 1 medium tomato, chopped
- ✓ 1 bunch of fresh cilantro, stemless and chopped

Ingredients:

- ✓ 1 red onion, chopped Juice of 1 large lime
- ✓ 3 tablespoons Dijon mustard
- ✓ ½ teaspoon fresh garlic paste
- ✓ 1 teaspoon Sumac Salt and pepper to taste

- ❖ Take a medium sized bowl and add the beans, chopped vegetables and cilantro. Take a small bowl and make the vinaigrette by adding lime juice, oil, fresh garlic, pepper, mustard and Sumac.

- ❖ Pour the vinaigrette over the salad and give it a light stir. Add a little salt and pepper. Cover and let cool for half an hour. Serve.

## 202) DEFINITIVE BUFFALO CASHEWS

| **Preparation Time**: 10 minutes | **Cooking Time**: 55 minutes | **Servings: 4** |
| --- | --- | --- |

Ingredients:

- ✓ 2 cups raw cashews
- ✓ ¾ cup spicy red sauce
- ✓ 1/3 cup avocado oil

Ingredients:

- ✓ ½ teaspoon garlic powder
- ✓ ¼ teaspoon turmeric

❖ Take a bowl, mix the wet ingredients in a bowl and toss with the seasoning. Add the cashews to the bowl and stir. Soak the cashews in the hot sauce mix for 2-4 hours. Preheat oven to 325 degrees F.

❖ Spread cashews on a baking sheet. Bake for 35-55 minutes, turning after every 10-15 minutes. Let them cool and serve!

## 203) DECISIVE RISOTTO WITH CAULIFLOWER AND MUSHROOMS

| **Preparation Time**: 10 minutes | **Cooking Time**: 20 minutes | **Servings: 4** |
| --- | --- | --- |

Ingredients:

- ✓ 1 cup vegetable broth
- ✓ 1 head of cauliflower, grated
- ✓ 9 ounces mushrooms, chopped

Ingredients:

- ✓ 2 tablespoons almond butter Sunflower seeds and black pepper, to taste
- ✓ 1 cup cream of coconut

❖ Take a saucepan and pour in some broth. Bring it to a boil and set it aside. Then take a pan and melt the almond butter over medium heat.

❖ Add the mushrooms and sauté them until they turn golden brown.

❖ Add the broth and the grated cauliflower. Bring the mixture to a boil and add the cream.

❖ Cook until the liquid is reduced and the cauliflower is al dente. Serve hot and enjoy!

## 204) SPANISH RICE CASSEROLE WITH BEEF AND CHEESE

| **Preparation Time**: | **Cooking Time**: 32 minutes | **Servings: 2** |
| --- | --- | --- |

Ingredients:

- ✓ 2 tablespoons chopped green bell pepper
- ✓ 1/4 teaspoon Worcestershire sauce
- ✓ 1/4 teaspoon ground cumin
- ✓ 1/4 cup shredded Cheddar cheese
- ✓ 1/4 cup finely chopped onion
- ✓ 1/4 cup chile sauce

Ingredients:

- ✓ 1/3 cup uncooked long grain rice
- ✓ 1/2 pound lean ground beef
- ✓ 1/2 teaspoon salt
- ✓ 1/2 teaspoon brown sugar
- ✓ 1/2 pinch ground black pepper
- ✓ 1/2 cup water
- ✓ 1/2 (14.5 ounce) canned tomatoes
- ✓ 1 tablespoon chopped fresh cilantro

❖ Place a nonstick saucepan over medium heat and brown the beef for 10 minutes while it crumbles. Discard fat. Stir in pepper, Worcestershire sauce, cumin, brown sugar, salt, chile sauce, rice, water, tomatoes, green bell pepper and onion.

❖ Mix well and cook for 10 minutes until blended and a little tender. Transfer to a baking dish and press down firmly. Sprinkle with cheese and bake for 7 minutes in the preheated 400oF oven.

❖ Bake for 3 minutes until the top is lightly browned. Serve and enjoy with chopped cilantro.

## 205) PEPPERS STUFFED WITH TURKEY AND QUINOA

| **Preparation Time:** | **Cooking Time:** 55 minutes | **Servings:** 6 |
|---|---|---|

Ingredients:

- ✓ 3 large red peppers
- ✓ 2 tablespoons chopped fresh rosemary
- ✓ 2 tablespoons chopped fresh parsley
- ✓ 3 tablespoons chopped pecans, toasted ¼ cup extra virgin olive oil ½ cup chicken broth

Ingredients:

- ✓ ½ pound fully cooked, diced smoked turkey sausage
- ✓ ½ teaspoon salt
- ✓ 2 cups water
- ✓ 1 cup uncooked quinoa

Directions:

- ❖ Over high heat, place a large saucepan and add salt, water and quinoa. Bring to a boil. Once boiling, reduce heat to a simmer, cover and cook until all water is absorbed about 15 minutes.
- ❖ Uncover the quinoa, turn off the heat and let it sit for another 5 minutes. Add the rosemary, parsley, pecans, olive oil, chicken broth and turkey sausage to the quinoa pan.

- ❖ Stir well. Cut the peppers in half lengthwise and discard the membranes and seeds. In another pot of boiling water, add the peppers, boil for 5 minutes, drain and discard the water. Grease a 13 x 9 baking dish and preheat the oven to 350oF.
- ❖ Place the boiled peppers on the prepared baking sheet, fill evenly with the quinoa mixture and bake. Bake for 15 minutes.

## 206) YANGCHOW CHINESE STYLE FRIED RICE

| **Preparation Time:** | **Cooking Time:** 20 minutes | **Servings:** 4 |
|---|---|---|

Ingredients:

- ✓ 4 cups cold cooked rice
- ✓ 1/2 cup peas 1 medium yellow onion, diced
- ✓ 5 tablespoons olive oil
- ✓ 4 ounces frozen medium shrimp, thawed, shelled, hulled and finely chopped

Ingredients:

- ✓ 6 ounces roasted pork
- ✓ 3 large eggs Salt and freshly ground black pepper
- ✓ 1/2 teaspoon cornstarch

Directions:

- ❖ Combine salt and ground black pepper and 1/2 tablespoon cornstarch, coat shrimp with it. Shred the roasted pork. Beat the eggs and set aside.
- ❖ Sauté shrimp in a wok over high heat with 1 tablespoon heated oil until pink, about 3 minutes. Set the shrimp aside and briefly sauté the roasted pork.

- ❖ Remove both from the skillet. In the same skillet, sauté onion until soft, stir in peas and cook until bright green. Remove both from the skillet. Add 2 tablespoons oil to the same skillet, add cooked rice.
- ❖ Stir and separate individual grains. Add beaten eggs, stir in rice. Add roasted pork, shrimp, vegetables and onion. Mix everything together. Season with salt and pepper to taste.

## 207) MOROCCAN SPICY COUSCOUS

| **Preparation Time**: 25 minutes | **Cooking Time**: | **Servings: 4** |
|---|---|---|

Ingredients:

- ✓ 1 cup instant couscous
- ✓ 2 tablespoons dried apricots, chopped
- ✓ 2 tablespoons dried raisins
- ✓ 2 tablespoons olive oil
- ✓ ½ onion, chopped
- ✓ 1 orange, squeezed and peeled

Ingredients:

- ✓ ¼ teaspoon paprika
- ✓ ¼ teaspoon turmeric
- ✓ ½ teaspoon garlic powder
- ✓ ½ teaspoon ground cumin
- ✓ ¼ teaspoon ground cinnamon Salt and black pepper to taste

❖ Heat the olive oil in a saucepan over medium heat and sauté the onion for 3 minutes. Add the orange juice, orange zest, garlic powder, cumin, salt, paprika, turmeric, cinnamon, black pepper and 2 cups of water and bring to a boil.

❖ Stir in the apricots, couscous and raisins. Remove from heat and let stand covered for 5 minutes. Fluff up the couscous with a fork. Serve.

## 208) RICE BOWL WITH VEGETABLES

| **Preparation Time**: 25 minutes | **Cooking Time**: | **Servings: 4** |
|---|---|---|

Ingredients:

- ✓ 12 ounces chopped broccoli
- ✓ 3 cups fresh spinach
- ✓ 1 red pepper, seeded and chopped
- ✓ 1 ½ cups cooked brown rice
- ✓ 2 tablespoons olive oil

Ingredients:

- ✓ 1 onion, chopped
- ✓ 1 clove garlic, chopped
- ✓ 1 orange, squeezed and peeled
- ✓ 1 cup vegetable broth Salt and black pepper to taste

❖ Heat the olive oil in a skillet over medium heat and sauté the onion for 5 minutes, then add the broccoli cuts and cook for 4-5 minutes until tender.

❖ Sauté the garlic and red pepper for 30 seconds. Pour in the orange zest, orange juice, broth, salt and pepper and bring to a boil.

❖ Add rice and spinach and cook for 4 minutes until liquid is reduced. Serve.

## 209) ITALIAN CANNELLINI BEANS WITH EGG NODDLES

| **Preparation Time**: 20 minutes | **Cooking Time**: | **Servings: 4** |
|---|---|---|

Ingredients:

- ✓ 12 ounces egg noodles
- ✓ 1 can be diced tomato
- ✓ 1 can be Cannellini beans, drained
- ✓ ½ cup heavy cream
- ✓ 1 cup vegetable broth
- ✓ 2 cloves garlic, minced
- ✓ 1 onion, chopped

Ingredients:

- ✓ 3 tablespoons olive oil 1 cup spinach, chopped
- ✓ 1 teaspoon dill
- ✓ 1 teaspoon thyme
- ✓ ½ teaspoon red pepper, crushed
- ✓ 1 lemon, squeezed and peeled
- ✓ 1 tablespoon fresh basil leaves, chopped

❖ Boil the egg noodles in plenty of salted water for 6 minutes or until al dente. Drain and set aside. Heat the olive oil in a saucepan over medium heat. Add the onion and garlic and cook for 3 minutes.

❖ Add the dill, thyme, and red pepper for 1 minute. Add the spinach, vermicelli, vegetable stock and tomatoes. Bring to a boil, cover and lower the heat. Cook for 5-7 minutes.

❖ Place the beans in and cook until heated through. Combine the heavy cream, lemon juice, lemon zest and basil. Serve the dish garnished with parsley and the creamy lemon sauce on the side.

| 210) | BLACK CABBAGE AND SPELT PILAF WITH PEAS | |
|---|---|---|
| **Preparation Time**: 50 minutes | **Cooking Time**: | **Servings**: 4 |

Ingredients:

- ✓ 1 cup green peas
- ✓ 4 cups kale, chopped
- ✓ ½ cup hummus
- ✓ ½ cup shallots, sliced
- ✓ 1 clove garlic, chopped
- ✓ 1 cup farro
- ✓ 2 cups water

Ingredients:

- ✓ 1 cup chopped tomatoes
- ✓ 1 tablespoon tomato paste
- ✓ 1 teaspoon cumin
- ✓ ½ teaspoon oregano
- ✓ 2 tablespoons fresh cilantro, chopped
- ✓ 2 tablespoons olive oil Salt and black pepper to taste

Directions:

- ❖ Heat the olive oil in a skillet over medium heat. Add the scallions and sauté until tender. Add the garlic, cumin and oregano and cook for another 30 seconds.

- ❖ Add the farro, water, chopped tomatoes and tomato paste. Bring to a boil, then lower the heat and simmer for 30-40 minutes. Add the peas, kale, salt and black pepper.
- ❖ Let stand covered for 8 minutes. Serve topped with hummus and cilantro.

# Chapter 3. DINNER

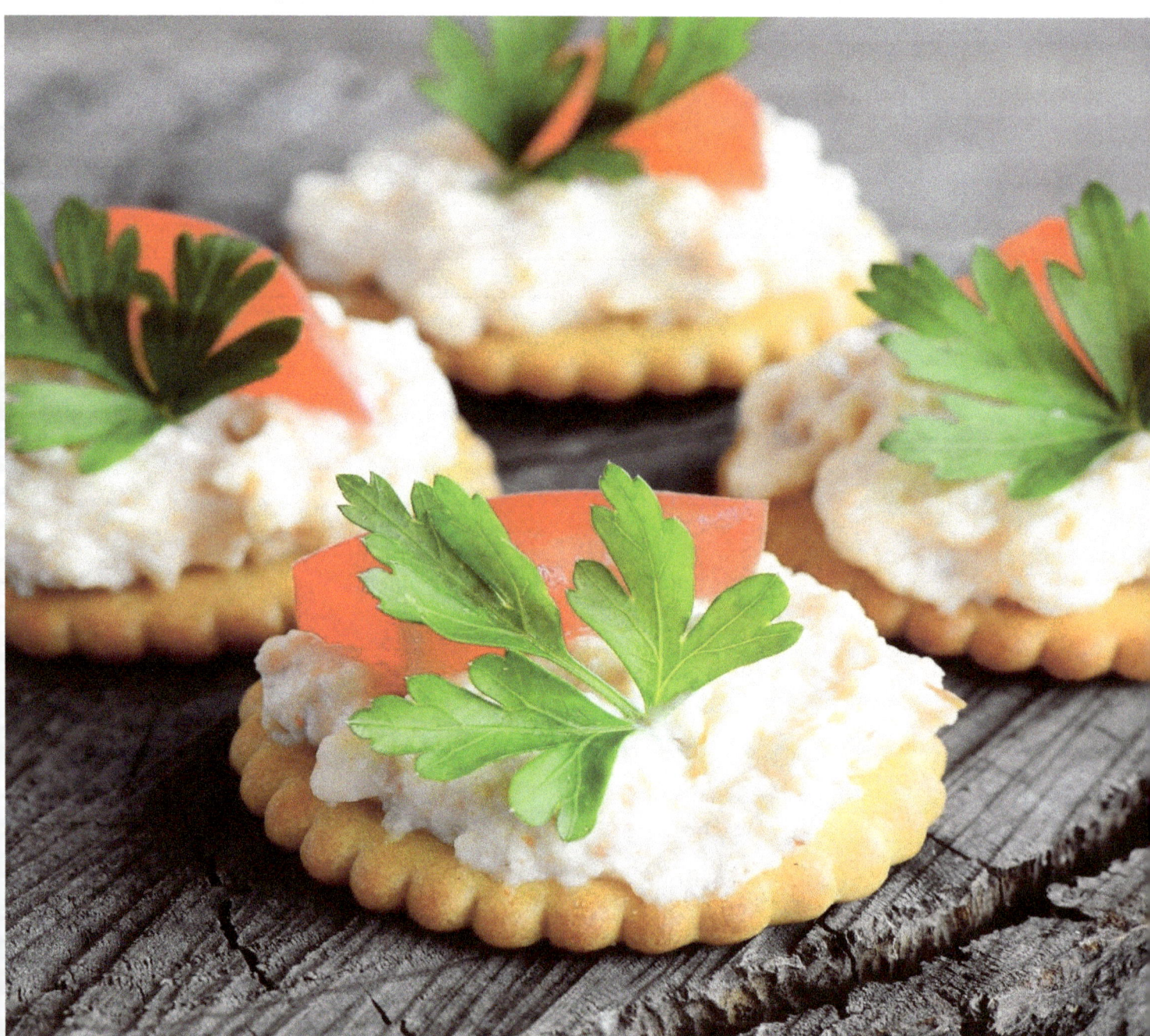

## 211) SPANISH RICE WITH CHICKEN

| **Preparation Time**: 50 minutes | **Cooking Time:** | **Servings: 4** |
| --- | --- | --- |

Ingredients:

- ✓ 1 pound chicken thighs, skinless
- ✓ 1 cup arroz bomba (Spanish rice), rinsed
- ✓ 2 cups chicken broth
- ✓ ½ cup spring onions, chopped
- ✓ ½ red bell bell pepper, thinly sliced
- ✓ ¼ cup tomato paste

Ingredients:

- ✓ 2 cloves garlic, minced
- ✓ ¼ cup white wine
- ✓ ½ teaspoon sweet paprika
- ✓ ¼ teaspoon turmeric
- ✓ ½ teaspoon dried basil
- ✓ ½ teaspoon dried tarragon
- ✓ 2 tablespoons Aioli olive oil, for garnish Salt and black pepper to taste

❖ Heat olive oil in a saucepan over medium heat and sauté chicken for 8-10 minutes. Remove to a plate to cool. Add the spring onions, bell bell pepper and garlic to the casserole and cook for 3 minutes.

❖ Pour in the white wine to scrape up any bits from the bottom. Discard the chicken bones and shred with a fork. Return to the casserole and sprinkle with salt, black pepper, paprika, turmeric, tarragon and basil.

❖ Add the rice, tomato paste and chicken stock. Cook covered for about 20 minutes. Serve garnished with the aioli.

## 212) LIMA BEAN STEW

| **Preparation Time**: 70 minutes | **Cooking Time:** | **Servings: 4** |
| --- | --- | --- |

Ingredients:

- ✓ 2 tablespoons olive oil
- ✓ 3 tomatoes, diced
- ✓ 1 yellow onion, chopped
- ✓ 1 celery stalk, chopped
- ✓ 2 tablespoons parsley, chopped
- ✓ 2 cloves garlic, chopped

Ingredients:

- ✓ 1 cup lima beans, soaked
- ✓ 1 teaspoon paprika
- ✓ 1 teaspoon dried oregano
- ✓ ½ teaspoon dried thyme Salt and black pepper to taste

❖ Cover lima beans with water in a pot and place over medium heat. Bring to a boil and cook for 30 minutes.

❖ Drain and set aside. Heat the olive oil in the pot over medium heat and cook the onion and garlic for 3 minutes.

❖ Add the tomatoes, celery, oregano, thyme and paprika and cook for 5 minutes. Pour in 3 cups of water and return the lima beans; season with salt and pepper.

❖ Simmer for 30 minutes. Sprinkle with parsley and serve

## 213) CAPER AND BROWN RICE PILAF

| **Preparation Time**: 30 minutes | **Cooking Time:** | **Servings: 4** |
| --- | --- | --- |

Ingredients:

- ✓ 1 cup brown rice
- ✓ 2 tablespoons olive oil
- ✓ 1 chopped onion
- ✓ 1 chopped celery stalk

Ingredients:

- ✓ 2 chopped garlic cloves
- ✓ ½ cup rinsed capers Salt and black pepper to taste
- ✓ 2 tablespoons chopped parsley

❖ Heat olive oil in a skillet over medium heat and sauté celery, garlic and onion for 10 minutes.

❖ Add rice, capers, 2 cups water, salt and pepper and cook for 25 minutes. Serve topped with parsley.

| *214)* | MILLET WITH CHILLI PEPPERS AND ZUCCHINI | | |
|---|---|---|---|
| **Preparation Time**: 30 minutes | **Cooking Time:** | | **Servings: 4** |

Ingredients:

- ✓ 2 tomatoes, chopped
- ✓ 2 zucchini, chopped
- ✓ 3 tablespoons olive oil
- ✓ 1 cup millet

Ingredients:

- ✓ 2 spring onions, chopped
- ✓ ½ cup cilantro, chopped
- ✓ 1 teaspoon chili paste
- ✓ ½ cup lemon juice Salt and black pepper to taste

Directions:

- ❖ Heat olive oil in a skillet over medium heat and sauté millet for 1-2 minutes. Pour in 2 cups of water, salt and pepper and bring to a boil.

- ❖ Cook for 15 minutes. Stir in spring onions, tomatoes, zucchini, chili paste and lemon juice. Serve topped with cilantro.

| *215)* | RISOTTO WITH BASIL AND PECORINO | | |
|---|---|---|---|
| **Preparation Time**: 35 minutes | **Cooking Time:** | | **Servings: 4** |

Ingredients:

- ✓ 2 tablespoons olive oil
- ✓ 2 cups chicken broth
- ✓ 1 onion, chopped
- ✓ 10 ounces sun-dried tomatoes in olive oil, drained and chopped

Ingredients:

- ✓ 1 cup Arborio rice Salt and black pepper to taste
- ✓ 1 cup Pecorino cheese, grated
- ✓ ¼ cup basil leaves, chopped

Directions:

- ❖ Heat the olive oil in a skillet over medium heat and cook the onion and sun-dried tomatoes for 5 minutes.

- ❖ Add the rice, chicken broth, salt, pepper and basil and bring to a boil. Cook for 20 minutes. Add the pecorino cheese and serve.

| *216)* | PORK WITH THYME AND RICE | | |
|---|---|---|---|
| **Preparation Time**: 8 hours and 10 minutes | **Cooking Time:** | | **Servings:** |

Ingredients:

- ✓ 3 tablespoons olive oil
- ✓ 2 pounds pork loin, sliced
- ✓ 1 cup chicken broth
- ✓ ½ tablespoon chili powder

Ingredients:

- ✓ 2 tablespoons thyme, dried
- ✓ ½ tablespoon garlic powder Salt and black pepper to taste
- ✓ 2 cups rice, cooked

- ❖ Put the pork, chicken broth, oil, chili powder, garlic powder, salt and pepper in your slow cooker.

- ❖ Cover with the lid and cook for 8 hours on Low. Divide pork among plates with a side of rice and garnish with sage to serve.

## 217) COUSCOUS WITH FETA CHEESE, CABBAGE AND CUCUMBER

| **Preparation Time**: 20 minutes | **Cooking Time**: | **Servings**: 4 |
|---|---|---|

Ingredients:

- ✓ 2 tablespoons olive oil
- ✓ 1 cup couscous
- ✓ 1 cup cabbage, chopped
- ✓ 1 tablespoon parsley, chopped
- ✓ 3 spring onions, chopped

Ingredients:

- ✓ 1 cucumber, chopped
- ✓ 1 pinch allspice
- ✓ ½ lemon, juice and zest
- ✓ 4 ounces feta cheese, crumbled

❖ In a bowl, place the couscous and cover with hot water. Let stand for 10 minutes and mash.

❖ Heat the olive oil in a skillet over medium heat and sauté the onions and allspice for 3 minutes.

❖ Add the remaining ingredients and cook for another 5-6 minutes.

## 218) HOT VEGETARIAN TWO BEAN CASSOULET

| **Preparation Time**: 40 minutes | **Cooking Time**: | **Servings**: 4 |
|---|---|---|

Ingredients:

- ✓ 1 cup canned pinto beans, drained
- ✓ 1 cup canned kidney beans, drained
- ✓ 2 red peppers, seeded and chopped
- ✓ 1 onion, chopped 1 celery stalk, chopped
- ✓ 2 garlic cloves, chopped

Ingredients:

- ✓ 1 can crushed tomatoes
- ✓ 2 tablespoons olive oil
- ✓ 1 tablespoon red pepper flakes
- ✓ 1 teaspoon ground cumin Salt and black pepper to taste
- ✓ ¼ tablespoon ground cilantro

❖ Heat olive oil in a saucepan over medium heat and sauté peppers, celery, garlic and onion for 5 minutes until tender.

❖ Add ground cumin, ground coriander, salt and pepper for 1 minute. Pour in the beans, tomatoes and red pepper flakes.

❖ Bring to a boil, then lower the heat and simmer for another 20 minutes. Serve immediately.

## 219) ITALIAN BARLEY WITH ARTICHOKE HEARTS

| **Preparation Time**: 50 minute | **Cooking Time**: | **Servings**: 4 |
|---|---|---|

Ingredients:

- ✓ 1 cup pearl barley
- ✓ ½ cup artichoke hearts, chopped
- ✓ 2 tablespoons grated Parmesan cheese
- ✓ 1 bay leaf
- ✓ 1 sprig fresh cilantro
- ✓ 1 sprig fresh thyme
- ✓ 2 tablespoons olive oil

Ingredients:

- ✓ 1 onion, chopped
- ✓ 1 tablespoon Italian seasoning
- ✓ 3 garlic cloves, chopped
- ✓ 1 cup chicken broth
- ✓ 1 lemon, peeled Salt and black pepper to taste

❖ water. Bring to a boil, then lower the heat and simmer for 25 minutes.

❖ Drain, discard the bay leaf, rosemary, and thyme, and store. Heat the olive oil in a skillet over medium heat. Sauté the onion, artichoke and Italian seasoning for 5 minutes.

❖ Add the garlic and sauté for 40 seconds. Pour in a little broth and cook until liquid is absorbed, then add more, and continue stirring until absorbed.

❖ Add the lemon zest, salt, pepper and cheese and stir for 2 minutes until the cheese has melted. Pour over the orzo and serve.

| 220) | SPICY CHICKPEAS BOWL WITH FETA CHEESE | | |
|---|---|---|---|
| **Preparation Time**: 10 minutes | **Cooking Time**: | | **Servings**: 4 |

Ingredients:

- ✓ 2 cups canned chickpea beans, drained
- ✓ 2 tomatoes, diced 1 cucumber, thinly sliced
- ✓ 1 teaspoon garlic, minced
- ✓ 1 red onion, chopped
- ✓ 2 green chiles, chopped
- ✓ 1 red bell pepper, thinly sliced

Ingredients:

- ✓ 2 tablespoons fresh parsley, chopped
- ✓ 1 fresh lemon, squeezed
- ✓ 1 cup feta cheese, crumbled
- ✓ 1 teaspoon harissa
- ✓ ¼ chili flakes Salt and black pepper to taste
- Fresh mint leaves, chopped

Directions:

- ❖ In a bowl, combine chickpeas with cucumbers, garlic, onion, chiles, tomatoes, bell bell pepper, parsley, lemon juice, chili flakes, harissa, salt and black pepper.

- ❖ Adjust seasonings. Serve topped with crumbled feta cheese and chopped fresh mint leaves.

| 221) | SPELT AND CHICKPEA STEW WITH HARISSA | | |
|---|---|---|---|
| **Preparation Time**: 35 minutes | **Cooking Time**: | | **Servings**: 4 |

Ingredients:

- ✓ 3 tablespoons olive oil
- ✓ 1 cup faro Salt and black pepper to taste
- ✓ 1 eggplant, diced
- ✓ 1 yellow onion, chopped
- ✓ 14 ounces canned tomatoes, chopped

Ingredients:

- ✓ 14 ounces canned chickpeas, drained
- ✓ 3 garlic cloves, chopped
- ✓ 2 tablespoons harissa paste
- ✓ 2 tablespoons cilantro, chopped

Directions:

- ❖ Heat olive oil in a skillet over medium heat and sauté eggplant, salt and pepper for 10 minutes; reserve. In the same skillet, add and sauté the onion for 3-4 minutes.
- ❖ Add the garlic, salt, pepper, harissa paste, chickpeas, tomatoes, lighthouse and 2 cups water.

- ❖ Cook for 15-20 minutes. Add the eggplant for another 5 minutes. Garnish with the cilantro and serve.

| 222) | ORZO WITH CAPER PEARLS AND TUNA FISH | | |
|---|---|---|---|
| **Preparation Time**: 50 minutes | **Cooking Time**: | | **Servings**: 4 |

Ingredients:

- ✓ 3 cups chicken broth
- ✓ 10 ounces canned tuna, flaked
- ✓ 1 cup barley Salt and black pepper to taste
- ✓ 1 cup cherry tomatoes, halved

Ingredients:

- ✓ ½ cup chiles, sliced
- ✓ 2 tablespoons olive oil
- ✓ ¼ cup capers, drained
- ✓ ½ lemon, squeezed

Directions:

- ❖ Boil the chicken stock in a saucepan over medium heat and add the barley. Cook covered for 40 minutes.

- ❖ Brush the orzo and place in a bowl. Add the tuna, salt, pepper, tomatoes, chiles, olive oil, capers and lemon juice. Serve.

## 223)  PORK WITH RICE COOKED UNDER PRESSURE

| **Preparation Time**: 35 minutes | **Cooking Time**: | **Servings: 4** |
|---|---|---|

Ingredients:

- ✓ 3 tablespoons olive oil
- ✓ 1 pound pork stew, diced Salt and black pepper to taste
- ✓ 2 chicken broth
- ✓ 1 leek, sliced
- ✓ 2 bay leaves

Ingredients:

- ✓ 1 carrot, sliced
- ✓ 1 cup brown rice
- ✓ 2 cloves garlic, chopped
- ✓ 2 tablespoons cilantro, chopped

❖ Set your robot to Sauté and heat the olive oil. Place the pork in and cook for 4-5 minutes, stirring often. Add the onion, leek, garlic and carrot and sauté for another 3 min

❖ utes. Stir in brown rice for 1 minute and pour in chicken broth; return pork. Lock the lid, select Manual and cook for 20 minutes on High

❖ When done, quickly release the pressure. Adjust seasoning and serve topped with cilantro.

## 224)  COUSCOUS OF FETA AND CHARD

| **Preparation Time**: 20 minutes | **Cooking Time**: | **Servings: 4** |
|---|---|---|

Ingredients:

- ✓ 2 tablespoons olive oil
- ✓ 2 cloves garlic, minced
- ✓ 1 cup raisins

Ingredients:

- ✓ ½ cup feta cheese, crumbled
- ✓ 1 bunch chard, chopped

Directions:

❖ In a bowl, place couscous and coevr with hot water. Let stand covered for 10 minutes.

❖ Use a fork to fluff it up. Heat the olive oil in a skillet over medium heat and sauté the garlic for one minute.

❖ Add the couscous, raisins and chard. Serve topped with feta cheese.

## 225)  LEMON CHICKPEAS WITH CARROTS AND CAPERS

| **Preparation Time**: 35 minutes | **Cooking Time**: | **Servings: 4** |
|---|---|---|

Ingredients:

- ✓ 3 tablespoons olive oil
- ✓ 3 tablespoons capers, drained
- ✓ 1 lemon, squeezed and peeled
- ✓ 1 red onion, chopped

Ingredients:

- ✓ 14 ounces canned chickpeas, drained
- ✓ 4 carrots, peeled and diced
- ✓ 1 tablespoon parsley, chopped Salt and black pepper to taste

Directions:

❖ Heat the olive oil in a skillet over medium heat and cook the onion, lemon zest, lemon juice and capers for 5 minutes.

❖ Add the chickpeas, carrots, parsley, salt and pepper and cook for another 20 minutes. Serve.

# Chapter 4. DESSERTS

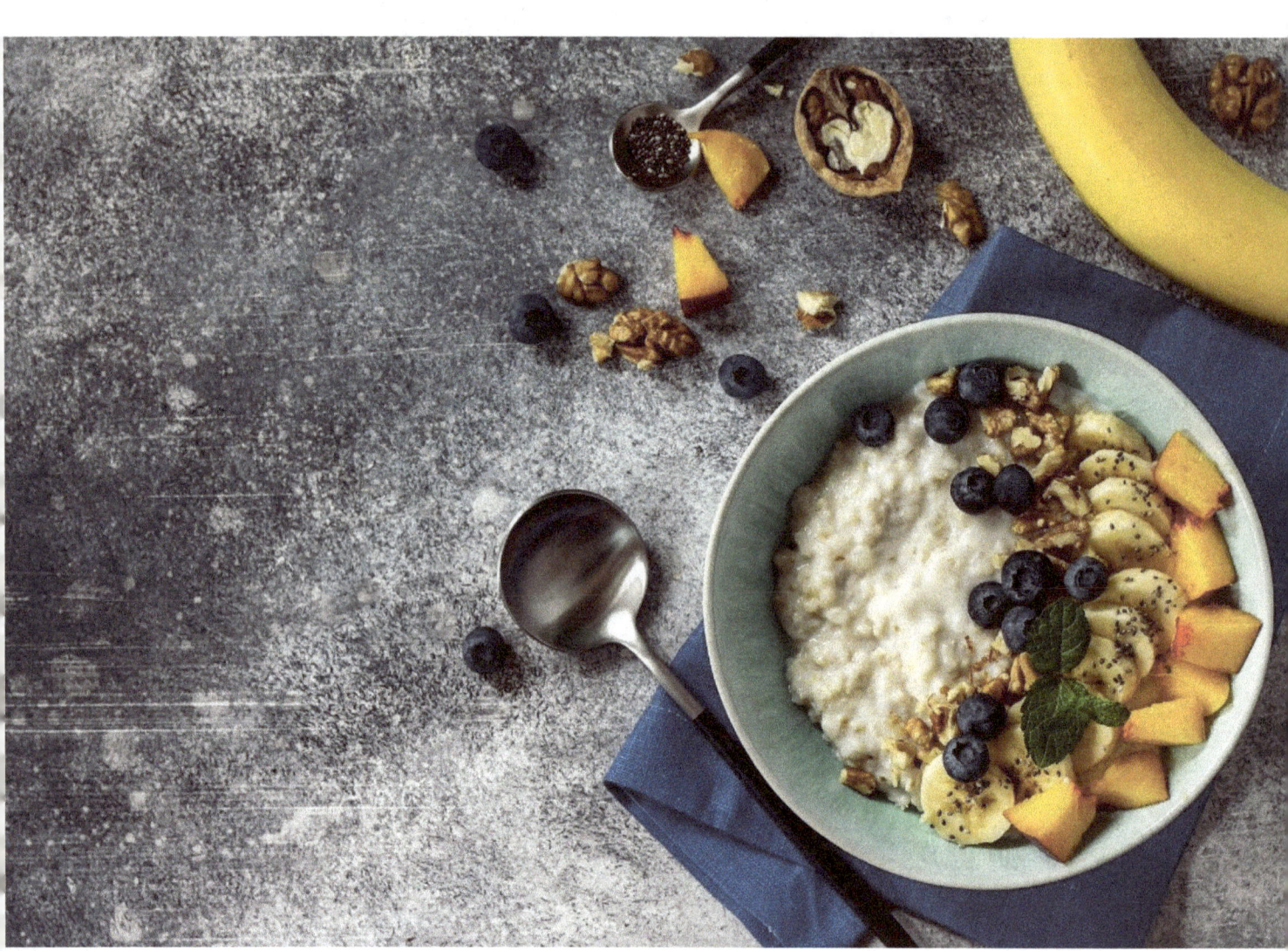

| _226)_ | STICKY CHICKEN WINGS WITH HONEY AND SOYA | |
|---|---|---|
| **Preparation Time**: 5 minutes | **Cooking Time:** 8 hours | **Servings: 6** |

Ingredients:

- ✓ ¼ cup of honey
- ✓ ¼ cup low-sodium soy sauce
- ✓ Juice of 1 orange
- ✓ 1 tablespoon fresh grated ginger

Ingredients:

- ✓ 1 teaspoon garlic powder
- ✓ 2 pounds (907 g) of chicken wings
- ✓ 1 teaspoon of sesame seeds
- ✓ 3 shallots, thinly sliced

- ❖ In a small bowl, whisk together the honey, soy sauce, orange juice, ginger and garlic powder.
- ❖ Place the chicken wings in your slow stove. Pour the sauce over the wings and stir to coat them.

- ❖ Cover and cook on low for 8 hours.
- ❖ Serve garnished with the sesame seeds and scallions.

| _227)_ | HONEY SPICED WALNUTS |
|---|---|

| **Preparation Time**: 5 minutes | **Cooking Time:** 4 hours | **Servings: 6** |
|---|---|---|

Ingredients:

- ✓ 2 spoons of honey
- ✓ 1 tablespoon of olive oil
- ✓ Zest of 1 orange
- ✓ 1 teaspoon ground cinnamon
- ✓ ½ teaspoon ground ginger

Ingredients:

- ✓ ¼ teaspoon ground nutmeg
- ✓ ½ teaspoon of sea salt
- ✓ ⅛ teaspoon of cayenne pepper
- ✓ 1 cup unsalted raw pecans (or other raw nuts of your choice)
- ✓ Non-stick cooking spray

Directions:

- ❖ Spray the pot of your slow cooker with non-stick spray.
- ❖ In a small bowl, whisk together the honey, olive oil, orange zest, cinnamon, ginger, nutmeg, sea salt and cayenne.

- ❖ Add the nuts to the pot over low heat. Pour the spice mixture on top.
- ❖ Cover and cook on low for 4 hours.
- ❖ Turn off the pot to a simmer. Uncover and let the nuts cool and harden for 2 hours, stirring occasionally to keep the nuts coated.

| _228)_ | CRISPY ROASTED EDAMAME |
|---|---|

| **Preparation Time**: 5 minutes | **Cooking Time:** 25 minutes | **Servings: 6** |
|---|---|---|

Ingredients:

- ✓ 1 (12-ounce / 340-g) bag of frozen, shelled edamame
- ✓ 1 tablespoon of olive oil
- ✓ ½ teaspoon of freshly ground black pepper

Ingredients:

- ✓ ½ teaspoon of onion powder
- ✓ ½ teaspoon of garlic powder
- ✓ 2 or 3 tablespoons of parmesan cheese (optional)

Directions:

- ❖ Preheat the oven to 425ºF (220ºC). Rinse the edamame in a colander until the ice has melted and the beans are almost completely thawed. Pat dry with paper towels.
- ❖ In a medium bowl, whisk together the olive oil, black pepper, onion powder, garlic powder, and cheese (if using). Add the edamame and toss to combine.

- ❖ Spread the edamame on a baking sheet that has been lightly sprayed with cooking spray. Roast the edamame for 20-25 minutes (stirring halfway through cooking) or until the beans are lightly browned and crispy.
- ❖ Serve immediately.

| 229) | CINNAMON APPLE CHIPS | |
|---|---|---|
| **Preparation Time**: 15 minutes | **Cooking Time:** 1¼ to 1½ hours | **Servings:** 4 |

| Ingredients: | Ingredients: |
|---|---|
| ✓ 3 apples, thinly sliced crosswise, with seeds<br>✓ 1 tablespoon ground cinnamon | ✓ 1 teaspoon of granulated sugar<br>✓ ¼ teaspoon of kosher salt |

| Directions: | ❖ Line up the apple slices on the baking sheet and roast for 45 minutes, then flip each chip and roast for another 45 minutes, until dry and crispy.<br>❖ Once cooled, store in an airtight container or plastic bag for up to 7 days. |
|---|---|
| ❖ Preheat oven to 275ºF (135ºC). Coat a baking sheet with cooking spray.<br>❖ In a large bowl, whisk together the cinnamon, sugar and salt. Add the apple slices and stir to coat them evenly. | |

| 230) | FIGS WITH HONEY AND CHOCOLATE SAUCE | |
|---|---|---|
| **Preparation Time**: 5 minutes | **Cooking Time:** 10 minutes | **Servings:** 4 |

| Ingredients: | Ingredients: |
|---|---|
| ✓ 8 fresh or dried figs<br>✓ ¼ cup of honey | ✓ 2 tablespoons unsweetened cocoa powder<br>✓ ½ cup low-fat Greek yogurt |

| Directions: | ❖ Combine the honey and cocoa powder in a small bowl, and mix well to form a syrup.<br>❖ Cut figs in half and place cut side up. Drizzle with syrup, top with a spoonful of yogurt and serve. |
|---|---|
| ❖ If using dried figs, place figs in a small heatproof bowl. Add boiling water to cover. Let stand in the hot water for 5-15 minutes; then drain before continuing. | |

| 231) | PEACHES WITH RICOTTA AND LEMON | |
|---|---|---|
| **Preparation Time**: 15 minutes | **Cooking Time:** 5 minutes | **Servings:** 4 |

| Ingredients: | Ingredients: |
|---|---|
| ✓ 6 ripe peaches, pitted and thinly sliced<br>✓ ¼ cup of water<br>✓ 2 tablespoons of Sucanat, or other raw or brown sugar | ✓ 1½ tablespoon of lemon juice<br>✓ 1 cup low-fat cottage cheese<br>✓ 2 teaspoons of lemon peel |

| Directions: | ❖ In a small bowl, combine the ricotta cheese and lemon zest. Mix well.<br>❖ Divide peaches among four bowls. Top with ricotta cheese and serve. |
|---|---|
| ❖ In a medium-sized heavy skillet, combine the peaches, water, Sucanat and lemon juice. Bring to a boil, stirring frequently. Remove from heat. | |

| 232) | HOMEMADE HOT CHOCOLATE | |
|---|---|---|
| **Preparation Time**: 5 minutes | **Cooking Time:** 5 minutes | **Servings: 4** |

| Ingredients: | Ingredients: |
|---|---|
| ✓ 4½ cups low-fat unsweetened almond milk<br>✓ 5 ounces (142 g) dark or bittersweet chocolate (70% cocoa), chopped | ✓ ¼ teaspoon ground cinnamon |
| Directions: | ❖ When the chocolate is melted, add the cinnamon. Whisk vigorously and serve immediately |
| ❖ Heat the milk in a saucepan over medium heat until just below boiling point, reduce the heat to low and add the chocolate. Stir gently to incorporate the milk chocolate. | |

| 233) | PLANTAIN WITH HONEY AND YOGURT | |
|---|---|---|
| **Preparation Time**: 2 minutes | **Cooking Time:** 2 minutes | **Servings: 4** |

| Ingredients: | Ingredients: |
|---|---|
| ✓ 2 tablespoons of olive oil<br>✓ 2 yellow plantains, peeled and cut into ¾ inch thick slices | ✓ ½ cup of low-fat plain Greek-style yogurt, or other yogurt<br>✓ 1 tablespoon of honey |
| Directions: | ❖ Combine the yogurt and honey in a small bowl.<br>❖ Drizzle the bananas with the yogurt mixture and serve. |
| ❖ In a medium nonstick skillet, heat olive oil until shimmering. Add the bananas and cook until golden brown, about 5 minutes. Turn and cook for an additional 3 minutes. Remove from heat. | |

| 234) | CREAM CHEESE AND CHUTNEY ON TOAST | |
|---|---|---|
| **Preparation Time**: 10 minutes | **Cooking Time:** 20 minutes | **Servings: 4** |

| Ingredients: | Ingredients: |
|---|---|
| ✓ ½ cup chopped dried apricots<br>✓ 1 cup boiling water<br>✓ ¼ cup of currants<br>✓ 1 teaspoon chopped ginger in a jar | ✓ ¼ cup white balsamic vinegar<br>✓ 2 tbsp granulated sugar<br>✓ 4 slices of spelt bread<br>✓ 4 tablespoons of low-fat cream cheese |
| Directions: | ❖ Simmer for 20 minutes, stirring occasionally, until mixture begins to thicken. Remove from heat and cool.<br>❖ Toast the bread. Top with cream cheese and a thin layer of chutney. Serve. |
| ❖ Place apricots in a medium nonstick skillet. Add boiling water and let stand for 10 minutes. Add currants, ginger, vinegar and sugar. Bring mixture to a boil over medium-high heat. | |

| | | |
|---|---|---|
| **Preparation Time**: 2 minutes | **Cooking Time:** 10 to 15 minutes | **Servings: 4** |

### 235) QUICK CABBAGE CHIPS

Ingredients:

✓ 2 heads of kale

Ingredients:

✓ 2 tablespoons of olive oil

Directions:

❖ Preheat the oven to 325ºF (163ºC).

❖ Cut the cabbage into pieces, removing the tough stems, and place in a medium bowl. Add the olive oil.

❖ Using your hands, massage the olive oil into the cabbage. When the cabbage is shiny, spread it out on a baking sheet in a single layer.

❖ Bake for 10-15 minutes, or until crispy. Serve or store in an airtight container.

### 236) NUTELLA AND BANANA SANDWICH

| | | |
|---|---|---|
| **Preparation Time**: 2 minutes | **Cooking Time:** 0 minutes | **Servings: 1** |

Ingredients:

✓ 1 slice of spelt or millet bread

✓ 1 tablespoon sugar-free chocolate hazelnut spread or roasted hazelnuts

Ingredients:

✓ 2 tablespoons of sliced banana

Directions:

❖ Cover the bread with the hazelnut cream.

❖ Cover with banana slices. Serve.

### 237) CRUDITÉ PLATE WITH HUMMUS

| | | |
|---|---|---|
| **Preparation Time**: 20 minutes | **Cooking Time:** 0 minutes | **Servings: 6** |

Ingredients:

Hummus:

✓ 2 (15-ounce / 425-g) cans of low-salt chickpeas, drained, rinsed and lightly heated

✓ ¼ cup olive oil

✓ Juice of 2 lemons

✓ 2 or 3 cloves of garlic, coarsely chopped

✓ ¾ cup of tahini

✓ ¼ teaspoon freshly ground pepper

✓ ½ cup of toasted pine nuts (optional)

Ingredients:

✓ ¼ cup chopped flat leaf parsley

Crudités:

✓ 12 baby carrots

✓ 12 cherry tomatoes

✓ 12 jicama sticks

✓ 12 sticks of celery, cut in half crosswise

Directions:

❖ Combine the chickpeas, olive oil, lemon juice and garlic in a food processor and puree until smooth.

❖ Add the tahini and pepper and continue blending until creamy.

❖ If it's too thick, add a little water to thin it out. Place the hummus in a serving bowl. Add the pine nuts and garnish with chopped parsley.

❖ Serve with crudités.

| 238) | WHITE BEAN DIP WITH DILL | |
|---|---|---|
| **Preparation Time**: 20 minutes | **Cooking Time:** 0 minutes | **Servings: 8** |

Ingredients:

- ✓ 1 (15-ounce / 425-g) can of low-salt cannellini beans, rinsed and drained
- ✓ 1½ tablespoon of lemon juice
- ✓ ½ cup of low-fat sour cream
- ✓ 1 cup plain low-fat yogurt

Ingredients:

- ✓ 1 tablespoon of dried dill
- ✓ 1 teaspoon of cumin
- ✓ 15 sticks of celery
- ✓ 15 baby carrots
- ✓ 15 wholemeal crackers or pita slices

Directions:

❖ In a blender or food processor, combine the beans, lemon juice, sour cream, yogurt, dill and cumin, and pulse for one minute, until the beans have broken down and all ingredients are incorporated. Scrape down the sides if necessary.

❖ Serve with celery sticks, carrots and crackers.

# Bibliography

## FROM THE SAME AUTHOR

**THE VEGETARIAN DIET** *Cookbook* - 100+ Easy-to-Follow Recipes for Beginners! TASTE Yourself with the Most Vibrant Plant-Based Cuisine Meals!

**THE VEGETARIAN DIET FOR ATHLETES** *Cookbook* - The Best Recipes for Athletic Performance and Muscle Growth! More Than 100 High-Protein Plant-Based Meals to Maintain a Perfect Body!

**THE VEGETARIAN DIET FOR BEGINNERS** *Cookbook* - 100+ Super Easy Recipes to Start a Healthier Lifestyle! The Best Recipes You Need to Jump into the Tastiest Plant-Based World!

**THE VEGETARIAN DIET FOR MEN** *Cookbook* - The Best 100 Recipes to Stay FIT! Sculpt Your Abs Before Summer with the Healthiest Plant-Based Meals!

**THE VEGETARIAN DIET FOR WOMEN** *Cookbook* - The Best 100 recipes to stay TONE and HEALTHY! Reboot your Metabolism before Summer with the Tastiest and Lightest Plant-Based Meals!

**THE VEGETARIAN DIET FOR KIDS** *Cookbook* - The Best 100 recipes for children, tested BY Kids FOR Kids! Jump into the Plant-Based World to Stay Healthy HAVING FUN!

**THE VEGETARIAN DIET FOR WOMEN OVER 50** *Cookbook* - The Best Plant-Based Recipes to Restart Your Metabolism! Maintain the Right Hormonal Balance and Lose Weight with More Than 100 Light and Healthy Recipes!

**THE VEGETARIAN DIET FOT MEN OVER 50** *Cookbook* - The Best Recipes to Restart Your Metabolism! Stay Healthy with More than 100 Easy and Mouthwatering Recipes!

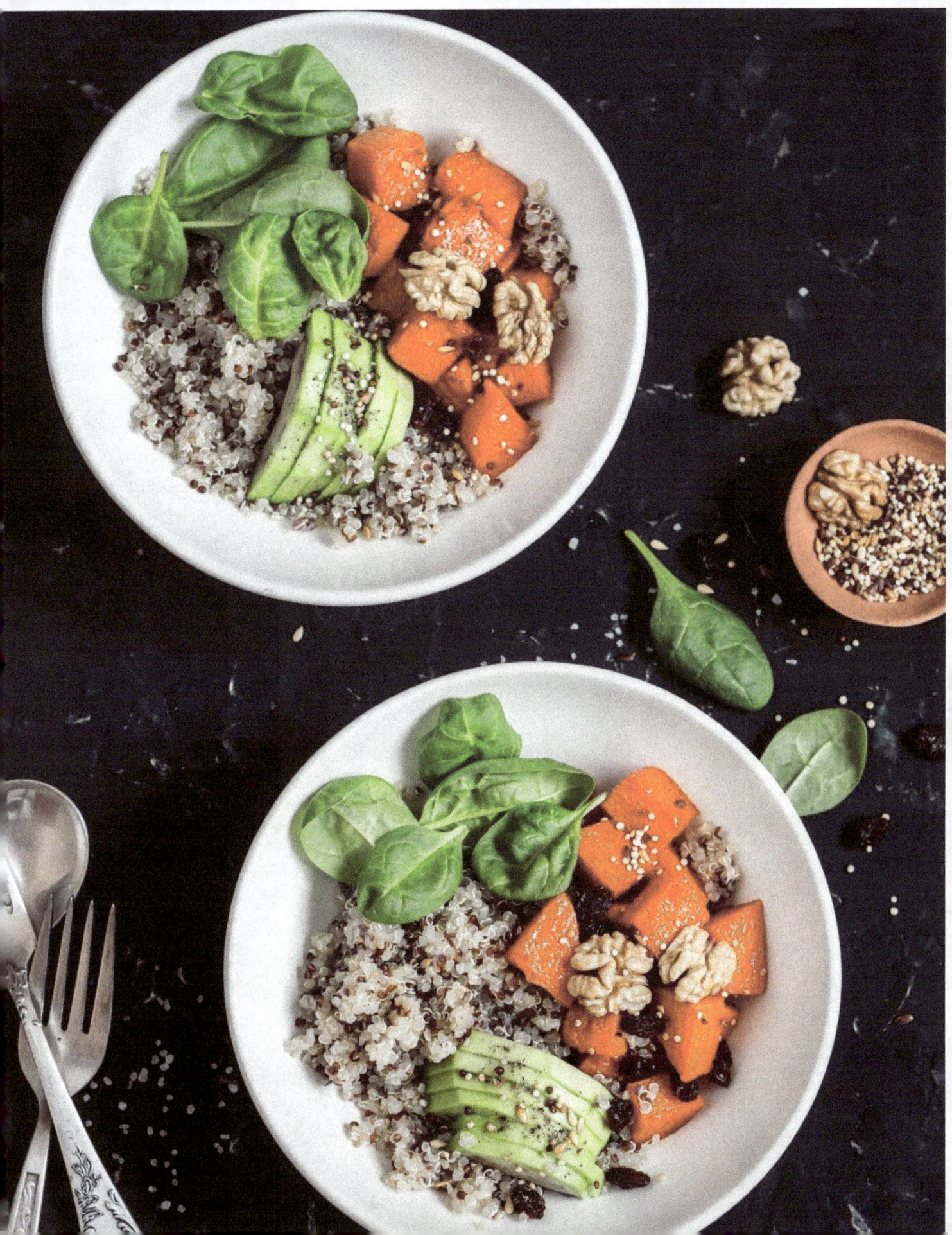

## Conclusion

Thanks for reading "The Dash Diet for Two *Cookbook*"!

Follow the right habits it is essential to have a healthy Lifestyle, and the Dash diet is the best solution!

**I hope you liked this Cookbook and I wish you to achieve all your goals!**

*Michelle Sandler*

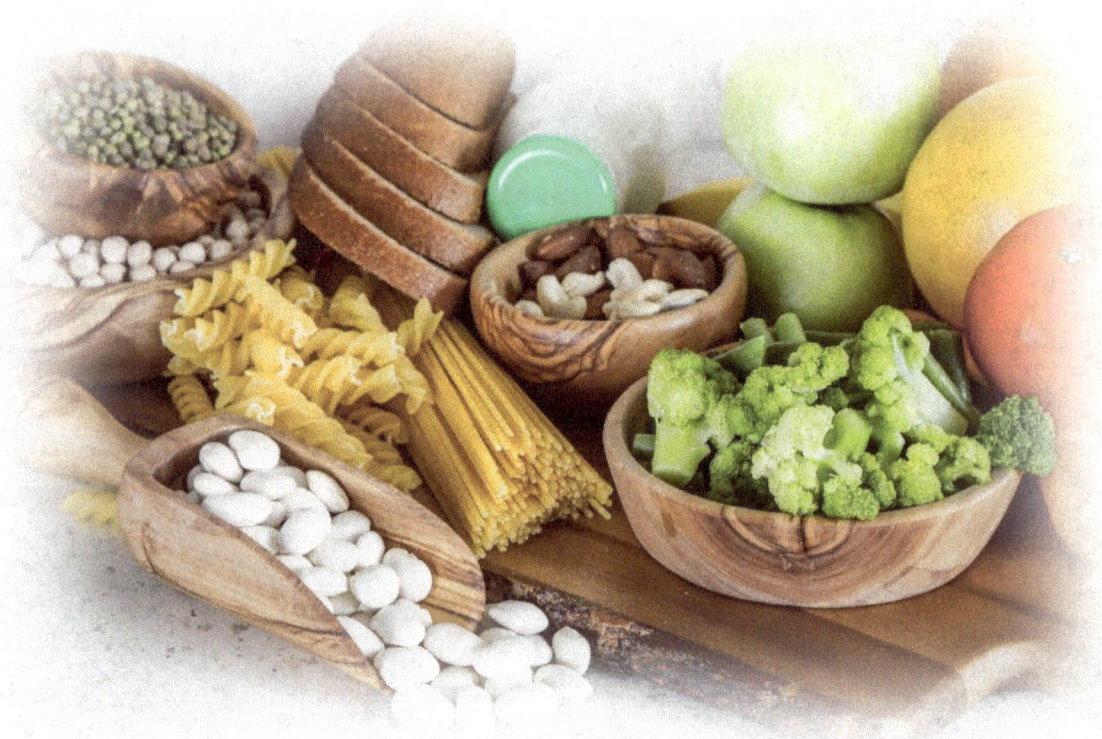